OPHTHALMIC THERAPEUTICS,

BY

TIMOTHY F. ALLEN, M.D.,

SURGEON TO THE NEW YORK OPHTHALMIC HOSPITAL, PROFESSOR OF MATERIA MEDICA AND THERAPEUTICS IN THE NEW YORK HOMŒOPATHIC MEDICAL COLLEGE,

AND

GEO. S. NORTON, M.D.,

SURGEON TO THE NEW YORK OPHTHALMIC HOSPITAL, OPHTHALMIC AND AURAL SURGEON TO THE HOMŒOPATHIC HOSPITAL ON WARD'S ISLAND.

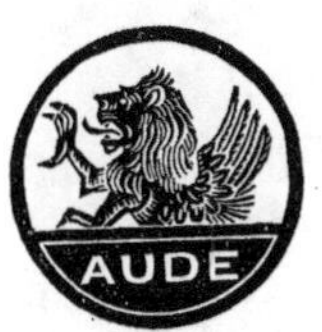

BOERICKE & TAFEL,

NEW YORK: 145 GRAND STREET. *PHILADELPHIA:* 635 ARCH STREET.

1876.

TO THE

NEW YORK OPHTHALMIC HOSPITAL

THIS LITTLE MANUAL IS

DEDICATED,

In appreciation of the facilities it affords for the relief of suffering and the advancement of medical knowledge.

PREFACE.

MATERIAL for this work has been accumulating for many years, especially since the adoption of the homœopathic method by the New York Ophthalmic Hospital.

When we first took our chairs in that institution, there were few indications for remedies associated with definite lesions of the eye; our cases were diagnosticated, and then carefully examined at all points for indications of the remedy, and from time to time groups of remedies have become associated with definite lesions and characteristic local indications recognized.

These local indications seem at times to be purely clinical or empirical, but they have always, or nearly always, been discovered while co-existing with positive and pure symptoms of the remedy, but they so often occur independently of the latter that they frequently assume a relatively greater importance.

Our knowledge of the pure effects of drugs upon the eye is unfortunately meagre, often quite indefinite and unsatisfactory; still, we have endeavored to keep to the standard, and have only permitted the introduction of clinical matter when the evidence has seemed to justify.

It is proper to explain that the plan of this work is substantially the same as that projected by Dr. Allen a few years since, and prematurely announced; the material then in hand has been augmented by the observations of Dr. Norton, the whole work written out by him and revised by us jointly.

Incomplete as we know it to be, we feel that its publication should not be longer delayed, and we offer it to the profession for most critical examination. *All the symptomatology given in this work has been verified;* when no authority is referred to, the editors are responsible, except when general reference is made to cases reported. Some observations may be ill-founded; many, we feel sure will prove reliable and contribute to the preservation and restoration of sight.

T. F. Allen, M.D.,
10 East Thirty-sixth Street.

Geo. S. Norton, M.D.,
36 West Twenty-seventh Street.

CONTENTS.

PART FIRST.

PART SECOND.

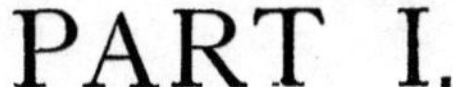

PART I.

OPHTHALMIC

THERAPEUTICS.

ACONITE.

Objective. The *lids* (especially the upper) *are swollen, red* and *hard*, with a tight feeling; worse mornings. The conjunctiva is intensely hyperæmic and chemosed, mostly towards the inner canthus. Inflammation extremely painful, so that one may wish to die. Lachrymation with local inflammations is very slight, if any.

Subjective. In the lids, *dryness, burning, sensitivenes to air.* Pressure in the upper lids, as if the whole ball were pushed into the orbit, causing a bruised pain in the eye; itching, smarting, burning in the eyes, especially worse in the evening. Sticking and tearing pains around the eyes, worse at night. The eye *is generally sensitive*, there is general heat and aching, worse on looking down or turning the eyes; feeling as if the eyes were swollen or as if sand were in them. *The ball* (especially the upper half) *is sensitive if moved;* feeling as if it would be forced out of the orbit (relieved on stooping); the ball feels enlarged, as if protruding and making the lids tense. Vision as through a veil; it is difficult to distinguish faces, with anxiety and vertigo. Photophobia.

Clinical. Aconite is the remedy for inflammations which are very painful, with heat and burning, as well as dryness. Inflammatory conditions, resulting from the irritant action of foreign bodies, as chips of steel, or stone, or coal, in the cornea, which produce dry rubbing of the lid over the ball, with injected vessels; also irritation caused by ingrowing lashes. *Catarrhal inflammation*, first stage prior to exudation; *chemosis* of conjunctiva, with pains so terrible that one wishes to die. In acute aggravations of *granulated lids* and *pannus* of the cornea, with excessive hyperæmia, heat and dryness, especially if the aggravation be induced by overheating from violent exercise, or by exposure to dry, cold air. In the earlier stages of violent acute *inflammations of the deep structures* of the ball, when it becomes sensitive to touch and feels as if it were protruding (rarely, if ever, called for after the exudation stage is reached).

In true sclerotitis, acute stage, with contracted pupils, sticking or tearing pains, photophobia, a blue circle around the cornea and violent aching in the balls (compare Spigelia).

The following case illustrates the good effects of Aconite in asthenopia:—A middle-aged man was employed to sort railroad tickets, to run through columns of figures and do other fine work by a dim light; in eight days he began to have a spasmodic closure of the lids and heavy feeling over the eyes, then his eyes would get very hot—"felt as though they could set a match on fire" or as after a lash with a whip. The conjunctiva of the lids was intensely red with constant winking and closing of the lids, could hardly force them open. The heat was always dry and temporarily relieved by cloths wet in cold water; vision normal; refraction normal. Aconite relieved these symptoms magically and allowed the man to continue his work (which he was obliged to do), till time enabled him to change his occupation.

Two cases of "total blindness," produced suddenly by taking cold, were cured with Acon.³ in water, every half hour one teaspoonful.—Hirsch.

AGARICUS.

Objective. The lids are half closed; swollen especially towards the inner canthus; *twitchings of the lids*, with contracted fissura palpebrarum without swelling. Twitchings of the ball, often painful; twitching of the ball while reading (especially the left); very little appearance of inflammatory action.

Subjective. Pressure and heaviness in the eyes, especially painful on moving them or exerting them by lamp light—with left-sided headache and involuntary twitching of the facial muscles. The bitings, itchings and jerkings about the brow and in the lids are very numerous in the provings. In the eyeball the sensations are mostly pressive and aching; the ball is sensitive to touch.

Vision dim, as through a veil, with flickering; reads with difficulty, as the type seems to move.

Clinical. Agaricus is of the greatest service in spasmodic affections of the lids and muscles of the balls, especially the internal recti. Chorea-like spasms of the lids, with general heaviness of them, especially if the spasms occur on waking or are relieved transiently by washing in cold water. In the *U. S. Medical and Surgical Journal* a case is reported of a child 2½ years old, idiotic in appearance, head top heavy, strabismus, numerous twitchings, soporous condition, who began, on waking, from a quiet sleep, to turn its balls rapidly right and left. Cured by Agaricus.

Cases of muscular asthenopia, with weakness of the internal recti, and consequent inability to keep the eyes fixed on reading (vanishing of sight), with pains around the eyes, soreness of the balls, twitchings and jerkings of the balls and lids, have been cured by this drug. Agaricus has also cured a very interesting case of anæmia of the optic nerve retina and choroid, with general tendency to chorea.

A lady suffered from muscular asthenopia, consequent upon uterine disorders and spinal anæmia (the spine was very sensitive to touch between the shoulders). She could not fix the eye long even on distant objects, could not converge the eyes (weak internal recti). She had sudden jerks in the ball itself, twitches of the lids, and at times in other parts of the body; the lids seemed heavy as if stuck together, but were not; she had been given prisms (which, though allowing binocular vision without effort, gave nature no chance of recovering herself), and had been under various forms of local and general treatment; after Agaricus the change was marvellous; within a week the eyes could be fixed on objects at ten feet without conscious effort, the unpleasant sensations had entirely vanished, and the patient was enabled to take up systematic gymnastics for the eye (initiated by fixing the eyes on a white object, while it is moved slowly right and left). The eyes have steadily improved, but the old pain returned in the spine, relieved only temporarily by applications of cold water.

Benefit has been obtained from Agaricus in myopia, dependent upon spasm of the ciliary muscle, especially if complicated with twitching of the lids.

ALLIUM CEPA.

Lachrymation excessive, especially of the left eye, with redness of the eyeball after frequent sneezing. Lachrymation (not excoriating) with coryza. The lachrymation is for the most part in the evening, in a warm room; the left eye weeps more and is also more sensitive to the light. Sensation as if something were under the lid, which causes a gush of tears to wash it out.

Clinical. Of use in acute catarrhal conjunctivitis, associated with a similar condition of the air passages, the lachrymation is not excoriating, though the nasal discharge is (reverse of Euphras.)

ALUMEN EXSICCATUM.

Clinical. This substance, first recommended by Dr. Liebold, has been employed with great benefit in trachoma, by dusting the crude powder upon the inner surface of the lids, allowing it to remain about a minute, more or less, and then washing it off with pure water. At the same time the lower preparations are given internally.

ALUMINA.

Objective. The upper lids are weak, seem to hang down as if paralyzed, especially the left lid; redness of the conjunctiva; the lashes fall out; small pimples or incipient styes on the lids; squinting of the eyes.

Subjective. Burning and dryness in the lids every evening, with pain in the internal canthus of left eye, with much dry mucus in the morning on waking. Agglutination mornings; the eyes burn on being opened, with photophobia; in the canthi itching; dryness and excoriation in the internal canthus; absence of lachrymation predominates and is characteristic. In the eye in general the sensations are: Burning, burning dryness, burning on waking, especially on looking up; pressure on the eyes (and balls), cannot open them; also photophobia.

Vision. Dim as through a fog or as if hairs or feathers were before vision. In the evening the vision is dim and eyes dry, so that she cannot use them.

Clinical. Alumina is indicated in chronic inflammations of the lids and conjunctiva, especially in chronic blepharitis. (Compare Graphites.) There is a dryness and smarting, without much destruction of tissue (ulceration), and without great thickening of the lids. Some chronic granular lids yield only to this drug (often administered by some locally as the aluminate of copper). The symptoms of loss of power in the upper lids are often met with in old dry cases of granulations; in these Alumina does good. The evening dryness and dimness of the eyes, with inability to use them, has been verified in cases of chronic dry catarrh. Alumina should be one of our most important remedies for loss of power of the internal recti (compare Ruta, Conium, Natr. mur.), and for paralytic squint.

A very remarkable case of "amaurosis," cured by metallic Aluminum^{200th}, was reported in the A. H. Z., vol. 54, by Bœnninghausen. The history details an inflammation attacking the eyes after childbirth, treated allopathically till "amaurosis" (*sic*) destroyed the left eye and began to affect the right. "The eye (vision) was most obscured in bright sunlight, and she could only make her way about the streets in the twilight; no colors before vision; everything black and dark; constant headache, worse towards evening and on motion; sweats easily. Bell. was first given to arrest progress of disease in right eye, which it did decidedly; then Con., "which acts markedly on the left eye;" then Bell. again, with effect to stop the clouds which began to re-appear over the right eye. She became pregnant and other complaints interfered with the eye treatment. In three months she complained of a yellow spot before the eye if she looked at white objects; this soon disappeared after a dose of Ammon carb.

After confinement she had various remedies and other treatment for a time, under which she became *stone blind.* She again improved under Sulph., Calc., Caust. and Sep., so that she could see her way about, but the eyes were very dim; the sleep disturbed by dreams, constipation and headache were complications. Having just received Alumin. met.[200], he dissolved some in six spoonfuls of water and ordered a spoonful night and morning for three days. The result was astonishing; complete restoration of vision (as good as formerly) and relief in other respects.

Compare. Dryness and burning in eyes, with Berberis, Natrum carb. and Nat. sulph.; dryness, etc., on reading, with Croc. and Arg. nit.; drooping lids, etc., Nux mos., Sepia and Rhus. Alumina lacks the moisture and tendency to crack, especially in the external canthus of Graphites. Alumina affects more the internal canthus, though not so predominantly so as Zincum. Alumina cases are usually relieved by washing the eyes.

AMMONIACUM.

Clinical. The following case is reported in B. J., vol. 2, by Buchner, as cured. Amblyopia occurring in a gentleman after a blow. There appears before his eyes as it were smoke, which, taking the flight of small birds, forms a large circle and is most distinct at twenty paces on a white ground. Generally smaller circles are present; in which case the smoke seems only an appendage to these circles. The appearance and motion of these circles depend upon the unsteadiness of the look and correspond to an appearance of congestion at the internal corners of the eye. The margins of the circles are always gray and become black on sudden motion. On first looking at an object, circles appear above the lens, but on looking steadily they sink to the middle and remain floating there. They are clearer in clear weather and dimmer in dark weather. Sometimes he also sees a black spot which becomes larger as night advances.

AMMONIUM CARB.

Eyes weak and watery, especially after reading. A large black spot floats before vision after sewing.

Clinical. Ammon. carb. is especially serviceable in cases of muscular asthenopia (affections from overstraining the eyes by prolonged sewing, etc.); compare Ruta, Coccul., Natr. mur., etc. On referring to Bœnninghausen's case under Alumina, it will be seen that he cured "yellow spots on looking at white objects," with Ammon. carb. So far as we know, this is a clinical symptom, but seems to have been one on which Bœnninghausen relied.

AMYL NITRIT.

Under the ophthalmoscope the veins of the disk were seen to become enlarged, varicose and tortuous; the arteries small but not abnormally so. Conjunctiva bloodshot. Protruding staring eyes.

Clinical. This drug has been found of great service in some cases of exophthalmic goitre; one case of which has been completely cured by the olfaction of Amyl nitrit. alone. (Compare Lycopus virg., Ferr., Spong. and Iodine.)

ANTIMONIUM CRUDUM.

Small humid spots in the external canthus which are very painful if sweat touches them; mucus in the canthi mornings, with dry crusts on the lids. Eyes red and inflamed, with itching and agglutination nights and photophobia mornings; lids red, with fine stitches in the ball. Itching in the canthi.

Clinical. This drug has cured or assisted in curing some obstinate cases of blepharitis which occurred in children. Its eye symptoms compare closely with those of Graphites.

APIS MEL.

Objective. *Lids much swollen, red and œdematous;* often everted; the upper lid hangs like a sack over the eye. Erysipelas of the lids; they are dark-bluish red, and so swollen as to close the eye, following severe pains; the swelling extends around the eyes and down over the cheek. The conjunctiva becomes congested, puffy, chemosed, full of dark-red veins.

Lachrymation hot, spirts out of the eye. Lachrymation, with burning in the eyes and with photophobia; with pains in the eyes on sewing evenings; with pain on looking at bright objects; with severe burning and sensation of a foreign body in the eyes.

Subjective. Burning, stinging and sensation of swelling around the left eye and in the superciliary ridge. Soreness of the lids and canthi, with agglutination; burning of the edges of the lids causes lachrymation. Stinging, itching in the internal canthi, or smarting of edges of lids. Stinging in the ball and pain across the forehead; aching pressing in the lower part of left ball. Fullness inside the ball, with flushed head and face.

Violent shooting pains over the right eye that extend down to ball. Smarting and sensation of burning in the eyes, with bright redness of the conjunctiva; very sensitive to light. *Stinging pains.* Pains on sewing. Most dreadful pains shoot through the eye in inflammations. Pains throbbing and burning. Pains aggravated by moving the eyes.

Photophobia. Eyes pain and are easily fatigued on exertion.

Clinical. The clinical record of this drug is very important, verifying nearly all its symptoms. It is especially applicable to inflammations, with burning biting pains; inflammations following eruptive diseases. Inflammations, with severe shooting pains, heat of the head, red face, cold feet, etc. Erysipelatous inflammations of the lids, with adjacent smooth swelling of the face, especially with chemosed conjunctiva, etc. Various forms of blepharitis, with thickening or swelling, such as incipient phlegmon, with great puffiness and stinging pains. (The following case by Dr. C. R. Norton shows its use in acute inflammation of the lids. Lids much swollen, red and blue, cannot open them, lachrymation, much pain, restless at night, *cold water gives great relief.* Grew worse under Acon.^{3}. Apis^{200}, cured speedily); chronic blepharitis, with thickening of conjunctival layer, so that the lower lid is everted. These swollen and everted lids often accompany chronic catarrhs with cornea troubles, which may call for Apis.

Some cases of ulceration of the margins of the lids and canthi, with stinging pains are reported. A very characteristic and aggravated case of lupus of the lower lid, which had gone on to ulceration, is reported cured by Meyer in A. H. Z., 63, 132.

Often the remedy for acute catarrhal conjunctivitis, in which there is bright redness and chemosis of the conjunctiva, with stinging pains.

Violent cases of Egyptian ophthalmia and ophthalmia neonatorum, with great swelling of the lids and adjacent cellular tissue are reported.

Various and severe forms of keratitis have been cured by Apis. Keratitis, with dreadful pains shooting through the eye, with swollen lids and conjunctiva; with hot lachrymation gushing out on opening the eyes; with photophobia (see Rhus). Pustular keratitis, with dark red chemosed conjunctiva and swollen lids. Ulceration of the cornea, vascular, with photophobia, lachrymation and burning pain; lids everted and often ulcerated on the margins. Scrofulous keratitis (parenchymatous), with dim vascular cornea, hot lachrymation, contracted pupils, etc. Opacities of the cornea have been reported cured, and even "staphyloma." (!)

Asthenopic troubles, especially affections from using eyes at night, causing redness of the eyes, with lachrymation and stinging pains.

A case of hydrops retinæ, with pressive pain in the lower part of the ball, with flushed face and head, was partially relieved by Apis but not cured.

The eye (and other) symptoms are aggravated in the evening and forepart of the night.

The character of the pains will usually serve to distinguish the Apis from the Rhus cases, which are objectively very similar. Apis does not seem to control suppurative inflammations of the deep structures of the eye as does Rhus, though the chemosis of the conjunctiva and puffiness of the lids might seem to indicate it; these cases are at first generally painless, and the external swelling is not bright red, as are the local and external troubles of Apis.

The burning hot lachrymation calls to mind Ars., but the discharges are not acrid and excoriating in Apis, though they feel burning hot; besides the Arsenicum cases usually present a well marked cachexia.

Kali bichrom. may be indicated when the lids are swollen and even œdematous. Kali hydriod. has also swollen red and ulcerated lids, etc.

ARGENTUM METALLICUM.

Margins of lids very thick and red. Violent itching in the canthi.

Clinical. This remedy has proved useful in some cases of blepharitis, relieving the severe itching of the lids and angles of the eye. One case of stricture of the lachrymal duct improved very rapidly under its use till lost sight of. (Compare the violent itching of this drug with Zincum, in which it is very marked in the internal canthus.)

ARGENTUM NITRICUM.

Objective. Ophthalmia, often with intense pain, abating in the cool and open air, but intolerable in a warm room. The conjunctiva both ocular and palpebral, becomes congested, swollen and infiltrated, with scarlet redness. The caruncula lachrymalis is swollen and looks like a lump of red flesh; clusters of intensely red vessels extend from the inner canthus to the cornea. Profuse mucous discharge in the morning on waking, with dullness of the head especially in the forehead and root of the nose. The margins of the lids are thick and red; the canthi red and sore.

(From the local application of this drug, most violent inflammation of the conjunctiva of the lids and ball ensues, with profuse muco-purulent discharge which is not excoriating to the lids).

Subjective. Boring above the left eye. Infra-orbital neuralgia. Burning, biting and itching in the eyes, especially in the canthi. Heat and pain in the ball on motion and touch.

Gray spots and bodies in the shape of serpents move before vision.

Clinical. Nitrate of silver has been very freely employed as an empirical remedy for various diseases affecting the conjunctiva and cornea; it is now, however, quite going out of fashion and being replaced by preparations of copper. It is very useful in blepharitis if the lids are very red, thick and swollen, especially if complicated with granulations, conjunctivitis or some deeper inflammation of the eye; in one case of ciliary blepharitis with entropion, caused from being over a fire, and ameliorated in the cold air or by cold applications, it effected a cure.

Nitrate of silver is not homœopathic to granular lids in the later stages, but is the appropriate remedy in the early stages of acute granular conjunctivitis, when the conjunctiva is intensely pink or scarlet red, and the discharge is profuse and inclined to be muco-purulent. Although these may be confounded with Euphrasia cases, there is a wide difference, more easy to recognize than to describe. In Euphrasia, the profuse discharge causes soreness of the lids and more or less swelling, the character of the inflammation is more acute and short-lived; as a rule, the redness is much less brilliant. In nitrate of silver cases we may, indeed, have very little discharge, only flakes of mucus when the patient complains of itching and biting in the eyes, and a dry burning sensation without real dryness. (Cantharis has intense heat and real dryness; Sulphur is very often indicated in these dry conjunctival catarrhs, especially if there be sharp sticking pains under the lids as if splinters were sticking into the eyeballs. Compare also Graphites, Natrum sulph., Nitric acid, etc.)

The greatest service that Argent. nit. performs is in purulent ophthalmia. With large experience in both hospital and private practice, we have not lost a single eye from this disease and everyone has been treated with *internal remedies*, most of them with Argent. nit. of a high potency, 30th or 200th. (Some have required other remedies, especially the form ophthalmia neonatorum.) We have witnessed the most intense chemosis with strangulated vessels, most profuse purulent discharge, even the cornea beginning to get hazy and looking as though it would slough, subside rapidly under Argent. nit. internally. We do believe there is no need of cauterization with it, for that method does not save all cases by many. The eyes *must be kept clean* with milk and water and not allowed to soak in the pus (this rule, indeed, is a good one for all similar diseases of mucous surfaces). The subjective symptoms are almost none; their very absence with the profuse purulent discharge and the swollen lids, swollen from being distended by a collection of pus in the eye or swelling of the sub-conjunctival tissue of the lids themselves (as in Rhus or Apis), indicates the drug.

Pterygium of a pink color was cured by a few doses of Argent. nit.—H. V. MILLER.

It has also relieved and contributed to the cure of diseases with destruction of tissue, as ulcer of the cornea, in one case with pains like darts through the eye mornings, better evenings; kerato-iritis with violent congestion of the conjunctiva; a vascular eroded cornea, with terrific pains from the vertex into the eye and with burning heat in the eyes. Coldness of the eye, with boring pain in the head and a sensation as if the scalp were drawn tightly, has been removed by Argent. nit. (Alumina is often indicated for coldness in the eye; Crocus has a draft of cold air through the eye; Berberis has a sensation of drops of cold water under the lids.) In the Argent. nit. cases we sometimes meet with trembling of the whole body and headaches.

An interesting case of paralysis of the accommodation is reported in which Argent. nit.^{6}, four times daily, worked a brilliant cure; also a case of retino-choroiditis successfully treated by this remedy.—WOODYATT.

A very interesting case, illustrative of the optical illusions of this drug, is reported by Dr. Liebold:—A young man was totally blind from cerebral disease, associated with loss of virility; was perfectly sane, but constantly complained that he seemed to see trees and people and green fields, etc., but everything was covered with *snakes*, writhing and twisting in every form; snakes over his body, over his food; snakes of all sizes everywhere; he would sit for hours and contemplate these snakes he seemed to see; sometimes he saw bugs. Dr. Liebold found in Berridge's Repertory, under "tortuous bodies," Argent. nit., among other remedies; it at once removed the snakes, but did not restore vision.

ARNICA.

The margin of the upper eyelids, along its line of contact with the eyeball, internally is painful when the lids are moved, as if they were too dry and a little sore. Cramp-like tearing or pressure in the eyebrow (left). Muscæ volitantes. Printing vanished and danced in a fog.

Clinical. Arnica has been employed with marked results in a variety of eye troubles resulting from blows and various injuries; sometimes applied locally (tincture diluted with water), and sometimes given internally. A few cases of subconjunctival ecchymosis, resulting from whooping-cough or from injuries, have come under our notice in which Arnica acted more promptly than Hamamelis; the relaxed condition of the blood-vessels and too fluid condition of the blood which predisposes to these hemorrhages in whooping-cough is often successfully met and corrected by Arnica.

Rheumatic iritis, marked by much lachrymation, photophobia and redness, with shooting and tearing pains in and around the eye aggravated at night and by warmth has been relieved; though Arnica can hardly be a remedy often indicated in iritis, unless caused from an injury; when it may be of service.

A case of traumatic mydriasis recovered very rapidly under this remedy.

Paralysis of the muscles from trauma has been cured, as in the following case of partial paralysis of the left superior oblique:—A man, 25 years old, after violent muscular exertion and injuries, saw double on looking down. There was an injury in left upper lid and a corresponding ecchymosis of the ball. Patient only suffered from diplopia and vertigo; he carried his head forward and to the right; was fearful of his balance, the ground seemed to waver under his feet; relieved by closing the left eye. The muscle recovered completely under Arnica.—Dr. Payr.

Asthenopia, as the following case will illustrate, has been relieved: A woman, 30 years of age, had been troubled for some time, after exposure in a cold bath with frequent muscæ volitantes. If she attempts to read the eyes pain and the print seems to dance in a cloud and vanish, so she must rub the eyes; there is a dull pain over the eyes even when not using them. Under the influence of Arnica she was cured.—Griesselich.

Retinal hemorrhages have been absorbed. A few cases are on record in which the sight was lost after a blow on the head, but was regained after taking Arnica, this might indeed happen without Arnica but it certainly seems to expedite absorption of clots.

ARSENICUM.

Objective. *Eyelids swollen and œdematous*, first the upper then the lower (this swelling is mostly non-inflammatory and painless); the œdematous lids are firmly and spasmodically closed, and look as if distended with air. Blepharadenitis ciliaris and ulcerosa; edges of lids very red. Continued trembling of the upper eyelids, with lachrymation. Conjunctiva inflamed; extreme redness of the inner surface of the eyelids. Lachrymation and discharges from the eye excoriate the lid and cheek.

Subjective. Suborbital pain on the left side with prickings as with needles, sometimes quite severe. Extreme redness of the inner surface of the eyelids, with an uneasy sensation, rather than pain, often obliging one to rub the eyes. Pain in the margin of the eyelids, on moving them, as if they were dry and rubbed against the balls, both in the open air and in the room. Burning on margins of lids. In the evening a feeling as of sand in the eyes, obliging him to rub them. *Burning in the eyes;* eyes hot, with burning, sore pain in the balls. Pulsative throbbing in the eyes, and with every pulsation a stitch; after midnight.

Photophobia. She appeared to be sensitive to light and often kept her eyes closed.

Clinical. Lids inflamed only on the internal surface; they are painful, dry and rub against the ball; they burn and can scarcely be opened. These symptoms are not uncommonly met with in chronic granulated lids, for which Arsen. is often indicated, especially if there are intense burning pains and excoriating lachrymation.

Pterygium, with dryness of the lids and the usual concomitant symptoms of Arsen. has been improved. (A. K. HILLS, S. B. HIGGINS).

In scrofulous ophthalmia, especially ulcers of the cornea, with soreness of the internal surface of the lids, which are swollen externally and spasmodically closed, so that opening the eyes causes intense, burning, sticking pain, especially worse at night; acrid tears gush from the eyes, the photophobia is excessive; opens the eyes well in the cool open air, but cannot in the house even in a dark room; the eyes feel as if they had no room in the orbit; throbbing pulsating in the eyeball and around the orbit, with general restlessness and prostration. Ulceration of the cornea recurring first in one eye then in the other, especially in young people who are anæmic (in one case when the eyes were better the feet were swollen).

A woman of thirty-five had ulcers of the cornea with chronic trachoma, with blepharitis which dated some years from the suppression of an eruption on the scalp which she described as scaly and very itchy. The cornea had become dim and dotted with small white scars from old ulcers, she had no lashes left, the lids were very sore on the inner margins; she had photophobia and various neuralgic pains. On the 12th of May she received one dose Sulphur 200th. In a week the right eye was somewhat better, but the left was much worse. The head is getting sore, with an itching moist eruption which forms a dry scurf; she complains of pains and restlessness at night; there is a twitching in the eyes as if they were drawing into the head, with burning heat, hot lachrymation and photophobia, with tearing pains around the eyes on looking at the light. Arsen.^{82m}, one dose was prescribed. In twelve days she reported wonderful improvement, no heat, no pains, no twitching, since the ulcers had healed the photophobia vanished; she received Sacch. lac. and continued to improve for three weeks, when a slight return of the photophobia necessitated a repetition of the dose; each dose acted about four weeks. She gradually recovered nearly perfect vision, with disappearance of the granulations and perfect cure of the eruption. Ulcer on the outer side of the cornea, with elevated edges, pain like the pricking of needles, excoriation of the external canthus, burning and sticking pains, promptly cured.

Vascular elevations on the cornea, resulting from ulceration, aggravated by opening and closing the eyes, with violent burning pains every afternoon.

Parenchymatous keratitis, with excessive photophobia; lies in bed with the face buried in the pillows, hot scalding lachrymation causes an eczematous eruption; paroxysmal pains; child fretful and obstinate (compare Rhus).

A very instructive case of keratitis punctata, with the following symptoms, is reported cured, by Schlosser:—Conjunctiva not hyperæmic, but with œdematous swelling of its outer segment; iris discolored and reacts sluggishly; posterior synechiæ, some exudation into the pupil, white punctate spots on the membrane of descemet, with burning pains in the eye, and upper part of the orbit, worse at night and accompanied by copious secretion of tears.

Kerato-iritis, several cases cured having burning pains over the orbit, worse at night, with profuse acrid lachrymation.

Iritis rheumatica, characterized by burning pains in the eye, worse at night after midnight, great restlessness and much thirst, has been cured. Has also been used with benefit in syphilitic iritis, in connection with atropine.

Retinitis albuminurica; Miss M. P., age 20, disease fully developed in both eyes; vision reduced in left eye to counting fingers at two feet; right vision $\frac{20}{70}$. Right ventricle hypertrophied; appetite variable; bowels regular; great thirst for small amounts; occipital headache of a pricking character; tongue large, dry and yellowish; menses too often and venous; breath oppressed, and pulse irregular. Cured in two months by Arsenicum 3d and 30th, and Sulphur 30th. Last report no albumen, right vision $\frac{20}{20}$, left $\frac{10}{50}$.—W. S. SEARLE.

Arsenicum cured a progressive choroiditis disseminata, which alternated with bronchial catarrh. When the eyes were better the chest was worse, and vice-versa. There was heat in the eyes, and burning in the chest, with dyspnœa, and a whole train of Arsenicum chest symptoms.

In A. H. Z., 44, 86, Dr. Schelling reports a case of suppressed catarrh, with headache and dim vision, so that only objects in the lowest part of the field of vision could be seen. (He walked with the head thrown back.) Everything above the axis of vision seems like a gray beard; the head was hot; the hair sensitive; paroxysms of most intense pains; Arsen. cured.

Doctor Stens, A. H. Z., reported a case of "amaurosis" with constant lateral motion of the balls, following a suppressed eruption, of which itching of the skin remained. Agaricus did not help. Sulphur, followed by Arsen. and again by Sulphur, cured.

Both Arsen. and Rhus are often indicated in scrofulous cases, but the paroxysmal character of the pains, the extreme prostration often present, the burning, sticking pains and the excoriating discharges may distinguish Arsen. The brilliant, red inner margin of the lids, and the dryness of their inner surface are very marked indications for its use in trachoma. The œdema of the lids, especially the lower one, is not at all like the puffiness of Apis or Rhus, nor is it dependent upon infiltration of the connective tissue, as it may be in Rhus, but is associated with the general cachectic Arsenic conditions. The nervous irritability, associated with the symptoms of Arsenic, is a very pronounced anæmic hyperæsthesia.

Arsenic cases are generally relieved by warm applications. They are very frequently periodic in their occurrence, commencing every fall, and often alternating from one eye to the other.

ARUM TRIPHYLLUM.

Clinical. A brilliant cure of catarrh of the lachrymal sac, with *desire to bore into the side of the nose*, was made by this drug.—C. A. Bacon.

ASAFŒTIDA.

Severe boring pain above the brows. Tearing pain in the forehead; dull pressure at the external border of the left orbit. Troublesome dryness of the eyes. Periodic burning in the eyes and pressing together of the lids, as if overcome with sleep. Burning in the ball from within outward.

Clinical. Asaf. is very useful in ciliary neuralgias, and from its power of relieving the intense boring, burning pain in the brows, especially at night, has arisen its very beneficial action in certain forms of deep-seated inflammation of the eyeball attended by these ciliary pains, as in iritis, kerato-iritis, irido-choroiditis and retinitis, especially if of syphilitic origin. The pains are usually throbbing, beating, boring or burning in character, either in the eye, over or around it; they are often intermittent, extend from within outwards and are ameliorated by rest and pressure (reverse of Aurum). It has relieved a sharp pain extending through the eye into the head, upon touching.

ASARUM.

Clinical. Asthenopia, accompanied by congestive headaches, has been cured. The eyes were worse morning and evening, when outdoors in the heat and sunlight; were better in the middle of the day and by bathing them in cold water.

ATROPINE.

About 9 P.M. eyelids felt heavy and difficult to keep open. Sharp pain under the right eye, with slight pain in the temples. Neuralgic pains, commencing under the left orbit, and running back to the ear, lasting perhaps ten minutes at a time, and then disappearing for fifteen or twenty; these have been noticed for several hours.

Clinical. In addition to the extensive use of Atropine for dilating the pupil, its use for the purposes of lessening the intra-ocular blood pressure in inflammatory diseases of the internal structures of the eyeball, and also in inflammations of the cornea and even conjunctiva, has lately come into vogue.

Its wholesale and empirical application for therapeutic purposes is most unwise and often unsafe, since we have few accurate data upon which to base a prescription of Atropine to cure (it should never be used when Belladonna is indicated, since Atropine does not comprise Belladonna).

It is a very happy provision, that the local application of Atropine to a healthy eye, almost always spends its whole drug power upon the peripheral nerve fibres of the iris and ciliary muscle; and that very seldom, indeed, do any constitutional symptoms arise. The instances of such marked drug affinity for accessible portions of the human body are, indeed, rare, or at least rarely recognized.

We have then a mechanical agent (as it were) for treating diseases of the iris. Neither Belladonna nor Atropine are often indicated remedies in iritis. Is then the use of Atropine to be commended? The necessary conditions for the successful treatment of iritis are above all:—First, Rest of the organ affected. Second, Isolation as far as possible from contiguous structures; in order to avoid adhesions of the iris to the surface of the lens. Rest of the iris can be approximately obtained by placing the patient in a perfectly dark room, and keeping him in a recumbent position. But we still have to deal with emotional effects, as well as the irritating actions of the inflammatory process. Darkness favors the dilatation of the pupil and consequent withdrawal of the margin of the iris from the lens capsule, but the inflammatory process supplies the stimulus or irritation which was banished with the light; and but little has been gained in sub-acute forms of the disease (often of long duration).

We cannot keep the patient constantly in the dark without detriment to his general health. Attempts of this kind have been attended with considerable damage to the patient.

In several years, we have seen no single bad effect from the use of a strong (4 grs. to the ounce) solution of Atropine, for dilating the pupil in order to examine the fundus; it is well, however, to avoid its use in all stages of glaucoma, as cases are reported of most violent inflammations following its use in that disease (though Belladonna does not seem to be at all homœopathic to glaucoma).

If an attack of iritis could be promptly recognized and met at the very beginning, before the exudative stage is reached (that is within 24 hours), there might be no need of Atropine, but if exudation has taken place, and the inflammation is violent, use immediately a strong solution of Atropine, a drop every four to six hours, it will not fatally interfere with the action of remedies though remedies may not act as well with as without it; it is, however, *in all cases*, the safest plan, for if adhesions take place, an iridectomy will usually be required. For sub-acute cases use a much weaker solution, one-quarter to one-eighth of a grain to the ounce; in any case use enough to accomplish the desired results, dilating the pupil; in severe cases, in which the congestion of the capillaries is enormous, and the iris cannot dilate, being so full of blood, use Aconite in frequent doses to reduce the hyperæmia, even temporarily; in rare cases of this kind, cupping of the temples would be justifiable as a temporary expedient, to enable us to obtain a dilated pupil; this being accomplished, remedial measures may be resumed and continued.

Its use is recommended for the relief of ciliary neuralgia.

AURUM.

Objective. Redness of the sclerotic; constant lachrymation; morning agglutination.

Subjective. Burning, stitching, drawing and itching in the inner canthus of eyes and lids. Sensation upon using the eyes as of violent heat in them. Pressure in the eyes and constant feeling of sand in them. Pressive pain in the right ball from above downward, also from without inward, worse on touch. Pain in the eye from blowing the nose.

Vision. *Hemiopia, the upper half of the field of vision seems covered by a black body*, the lower half visible. He cannot distinguish anything clearly, because he sees everything double, and one object is seen mixed with the other, with violent tension in the eyes.

Clinical. In blepharitis it is rarely useful, though sometimes called for, especially in syphilitic patients after the abuse of Mercury.

Several cases of trachoma, with and without pannus (especially with) have been greatly benefited, and there is probably no remedy in the materia medica oftener adapted to this condition than Aurum; the pains may be burning or dull in character, compelling one to close the lids, are usually worse in the morning and ameliorated by the application of cold water.

For corneal ulcerations and pannus-like thickening of the outer layer, no remedy is of so much value, especially in the cases of scrofulous ophthalmia, with ulcerations and vascularity of the cornea, with great irritability of the patient; great sensitiveness to noise; photophobia, profuse scalding lachrymation, eyes very sensitive to touch, swollen cervical glands, pains from without inward, worse on touch (reverse of Asaf.).

In interstitial keratitis and kerato-iritis (even in sluggish atonic cases), with an infiltrated cornea and fine interstitial vascularity, Aurum has proved itself of the greatest value.

In several cases it has hastened the absorption of deposits in the cornea, and cleared up opacities remaining after ulcerations or infiltration.

Iritis, (particularly the syphilitic variety and after the abuse of Mercury) marked by much pain around the eye, which seems to be deep in the bone, extends from without inward and is aggravated by touch, is relieved by Aurum.

Choroiditis, with injection of sub-conjunctival vessels, slight iritis, photophobia, pains in the hip, great craving for coffee and general feeling of malaise, was cured by this remedy.—Harvey Gilbert.

Has been recommended and used with benefit in paralysis of the muscles due to syphilitic periostitis.

The following case of "glaucoma" (?) reported by E. M. Pease, in M. I., is instructive. "Mr. J., æt. 24, lawyer, while reading was suddenly affected with partial loss of sight. Seeking medical advice, he was told that he was suffering from congestion of the retina and was put under the use of Mercury. After a few weeks of treatment, (being twice salivated) he lost his eyesight completely. January 14th, 1873. Received Acon.^{12}, first three times, then twice per day. January 30th. Could distinguish light from darkness; improved slowly to March 26th. Complaining of fulness over the eyes and floating specks in vision. He received Apis^{2c} and Merc. viv.^{30m}.

March 31st. His state was as follows:—"Feeling of severe pressure from within outward and from above downward, in both eyeballs, accompanied by dull, heavy aching, deep in both globes. On pressure, the eyeballs more tense and firm than usual. He saw yellow, crescent-shaped bodies floating obliquely upward in the field of vision; sees a little better on looking intently and steadily at an object, *though he sees no trace of the upper half of an object.* In the upper dark section of the field of vision, occasional showers of bright, star-like bodies, the lower half looks lighter, and he can distinguish color, light or dark. By gaslight a number of bright floating streaks and dots are seen; eyes better by moonlight and after active muscular exercise; pupils irregularly dilated; cornea dull, with loss of usual lustre; anterior chamber contracted; color of the optic nerve-entrances of a greenish hue, except around the periphery, which was yellowish white, with a slight trace of pigmentary deposit on lower outer edge of optic disk in left eye; the retinal vessels bent abruptly on their exit from the disk, and closely hugging the floor of the excavation, bent sharply upon the periphery of the papilla; central portion of retinal vessels strongly pulsating; large letters cannot be distinguished, he seeing only something black upon a white ground. Aurum was given in the 200th. After three weeks, patient was much improved, could get about the streets alone, being able to follow the cracks in a board sidewalk; the dark, half-vision, had disappeared, seeing as well the upper as the lower half of an object.

Five weeks from commencing with Aurum, everything looked blue and objects generally much lighter. May 5th. He received Aurum^{m}, but was shortly after lost sight of by removing to the West."—An. Record.

Hemiopia. A man, æt. 52, accustomed to drink whiskey every day, has complained for three months of a gradual decrease of vision. At first it appeared to him as if a fog or smoke lay before his eyes; to this, at a later period, black spots were added, and for the last few weeks he can only see the upper half of objects; their lower half seems to be covered by a black veil. Appetite poor; sleep restless and full of anxious dreams; is sad and would cry all the time. Ophthalmoscopic examination gives no clue. Thinking that it was due to the whiskey it was strictly forbidden. Aurum cured in four weeks, notwithstanding the patient did not abstain from his accustomed dram.—Baumann in A. H. Z.

Hemiopia, in which nothing to the right side can be seen, has been helped though not cured. But the form of hemiopia, to which Aurum is especially adapted, is when they can see nothing above the medium line, as the following cases illustrate. Some years ago a gentleman who had taken large quantities of Iodide of Potash, complained that the vision of the left eye had been failing for a year and a half; he could not see the upper half of a room or any large object, though the lower half was clear; no pains in the eye, objects seem smaller and more distant, has some black spots before vision, is always worse as the day progresses and better in the morning; twitching in the upper lid. On inquiry it was found that he had had syphilis ten years ago, but had not been recently troubled with any secondary symptoms, except that a large bursa-like swelling on the wrist has persisted a long time. Vision was $\frac{5}{200}$. Upon ophthalmoscopic examination there was found chorio-retinitis (chronic) with an accumulation of fluid beneath the retina, which settled to the lower portion of the eye and caused a large detachment of the retina. Vitreous hazy from infiltration. Right eye normal; refraction normal. Knowledge of the pathological condition here gave no clue to the remedy, and we were obliged, this time at least, to rely upon the symptomatology (as one should be always ready to do). The remarkable symptom of not seeing anything in the upper half of the field of vision, is, of course, the most prominent; in addition to the Aurum symptom, we may find under Digitalis, "as if the upper half of the field of vision were covered by a dark cloud evenings on walking." Digitalis, moreover, covers the pathological point, having been found curative in fluid exudations of various kinds; it is also worse in the evening, while Aurum is usually worse in the morning; still taking the history of the case into account, and the previous dosing with Iodide of Potash, Aurum 200th was given, under which he steadily improved, the haziness of the vitreous almost entirely disappeared, the inflammation of the retina subsided, and in one year the vision rose to and remained at $\frac{15}{100}$, beyond which it will not go, for the retina was partly disorganized and cannot be repaired with retinal tissue.

Since then, several cases of the same disease have been treated with Aurum, with almost unvarying success, though in some cases no improvement followed, and the remedy only served to arrest further progress of the malady. Many of these cases will be found to follow overdosing by Potash or Mercury, and perfect vision can never be expected from the nature of the tissue changes.

One singular case of a man, forty years old, was sent for advice. A large black, sub-choroidal tumor was found behind the lens in the fundus, growing from the inner side; he suffered no pain, but the symptoms of vision were those of Aurum, (the whole disease had only lasted about six weeks) vision $\frac{5}{200}$. After taking Aurum 200th, a week, vision rose to $\frac{5}{80}$; and in eight weeks more to $\frac{5}{60}$; since which time he has not been seen. It was probably an exudation tumor and may have been absorbed.

AURUM MURIATICUM.

Clinical. This is the form of gold, usually employed when we desire to use the lower preparations; its sphere of action, as far as known, differs little from the metal itself.

Several cases of keratitis parenchymatosa, cornea very opaque, traversed by a dense mass of blood-vessels in the cornea, proper (or not), and tending towards staphyloma, ciliary injection, some photophobia, and no vision, have been cured very rapidly by the first trituration of the muriate of gold.

Complete blindness, occurring suddenly after scarlet fever, with cold sweat, rapid, scarcely perceptible pulse, respiration rapid and unequal, abdomen burning hot, extremities cold and covered with sweat, is reported cured.—ALTMÜLLER.

BARYTA CARBONICA.

Redness of the conjunctiva, with swollen lids. Itching in the eyes. Sensation of a gauze before the eyes in the morning and after a meal.

Clinical. Has been recommended and used with success in scrofulous inflammations of the eye, characterized by phlyctenules and ulcers on the cornea, especially when associated with glandular swellings.

Cataract and morbus basedowii are said to have been helped.

Amblyopia, if caused by age, is removed by Baryta carb.—T. S. HOYNE.

BARYTA IODATA.

Clinical. Up to the present time no proving has been made of this substance, so that its sphere of action is hypothecated from its composition clinically, it has proved a great addition to our armamentarium. It was first introduced into notice as an ophthalmic remedy by Dr. Liebold, who says that it is especially adapted to diseases occurring in scrofulous subjects, in which there is great swelling of the glands, particularly of the lymphatics, which "feel like a string of beans everywhere between the muscles, down to the spinal column; they can be felt of all sizes and all degrees of induration; some may be suppurating, while others have healed with an ugly scar." It has been used very successfully in chronic recurrences of phlyctenular keratitis and conjunctivitis found in the above subjects.

Specific interstitial keratitis of both eyes, in which vision had decreased so that fingers could be counted at not more than four feet, complicated with enlargement of the cervical glands, which are hard and painful on pressure, is reported cured.—WOODYATT.

BELLADONNA.

Objective. The eyes are protruding, staring and brilliant. The eyes become distorted, with redness and swelling of the face; spasms of the eyes; the eyes are in constant motion. Lids puffy, red and congested; inflammatory swelling of the lower lid near the inner canthus, with throbbing pains, etc. Conjunctiva red, tumefied. Lachrymation, with great photophobia; total absence of lachrymation and motion of the eyes attended with a sense of dryness and stiffness; the conjunctival vessels fully injected. Pupils, (at first, or from large doses) dilated; (afterward, or from minute doses) contracted. The optic disk greatly deepened in tint, and the retinal arteries and veins much enlarged, the veins most markedly so.

Subjective. Eye dry, motion attended with a sense of dryness and stiffness. Pain and burning in the eyes. Feeling of heat in the eyes; it seems as if they were surrounded by a hot vapor. Burning heat in the eyes. The surface of the ball became quite dry, which caused a very disagreeable and uncomfortable sensation, which could not be relieved by winking or continued closing of the eyes. Pressive pain deep in ball when she closed the eyes; feeling as if the eyes protruded.

Vision. Dimness of sight or actual blindness. Every object in the room, both real and spectral, had a double or at least a dim outline, owing to the extreme dilatation of the pupils. Everything he looks at seems red. A large halo appears round the flame of the candle, partly colored, the red predominating; at times the light seems as if broken up into rays. Occasional flashes of light before the eyes; sparks as of electricity before the eyes, especially on moving them; large bright sparks before the eyes. Retina, insensible, he is quite blind. *Photophobia.*

Clinical. The use of this drug in inflammatory disease of the eye, is much more limited than is generally supposed.

In blepharitis, if the lids are painful and swollen like erysipelas, it may be useful.

In some forms of conjunctivitis (especially catarrhal in the early stages) with dryness of the eyes, thickened red lids and burning pains in the eye, it is the remedy.

It may be required as a temporary remedy in acute aggravations of various chronic diseases, as in granular lids, when, after taking cold, the eyes become sensitive to air and light, with dryness and a gritty feeling; or in chronic keratitis, when suddenly the eye becomes intensely congested, with heat, pains, photophobia, etc.; pains often sharp, shooting through the ball to the back of the head.

Rheumatic iritis has been aborted in the early stages by Bell., but the remedy is not often indicated.

Mydriasis, resulting from nervous headache, has been relieved.

Convulsive movements of the eyeball in the light, with terrible pressive pain extending through the whole head, ameliorated in a dark room, have been cured by Bell.; hence its use has been recommended in strabismus, due to spasmodic action of the muscles or when resulting from brain affections.

In orbital neuralgias, especially of the infra-orbital nerve, with red face, hot hands, etc., it is a valuable remedy.

Particularly useful in diseases of the fundus, of almost every kind and character. Hyperæsthesia of the retina, so often found in ametropic conditions of the eye, is often quickly relieved.

But in hyperæmia of the optic nerve and retina, it is especially indicated, particularly if dependent upon cerebral congestion and accompanied by aching pain in the eye, aggravated by any light; also in chronic forms of hyperæmia, if a red conjunctival line is very marked along the line of fissure of the lids. In some of these cases, as well as in some acute inflammatory affections, retinal photopsies are present, such as red sparks, flames, bright spots, lights, etc.

Its usefulness is not, however, confined to simple congestion of the optic nerve and retina; it is one of our chief remedies in inflammation of these tissues. A case of optic neuritis, in which the papilla was very much swollen, veins large, flashes of light before the eye and pains in the head; also a case of retinitis in a young lady (subject to congestive headaches, always worse in the afternoon): Retina very hazy and œdematous, appearing as if covered with a bluish-gray film, outlines of disk ill-defined, vessels large and tortuous, are instances in which Bell. worked rapid cures. Apoplexy of the retina, with suppression of menstruation, occurring in a girl, eighteen years of age, is reported by Payr:—She was subject to cerebral congestions, sudden heat of head, vertigo, burning and throbbing frontal pain, noises in the ear and illusions of vision, while the rest of the body was cold and shivering. Headaches increased, pulsation of the carotids became more severe, photopsies and then sudden blindness. Numerous apoplectic spots were found in the macula lutea, no change of papilla, pulsation of central vein; much active cerebral congestion and great photophobia. Under Bell. complete recovery of vision and absorption of the hemorrhages took place.

Has been employed in choroiditis, especially the disseminate form with great advantage. Bell. has wonderfully relieved the severe pains of glaucoma and afforded temporary relief; (glaucomatous eyes are exceedingly sensitive to the action of this drug and Atropine should never be used, if possible to avoid it.)

Several cases of amaurosis and amblyopia are on record, as the following cases will illustrate, in which the vision was restored by this remedy. Amaurosis of four years duration, occurring after suppression of the rash in scarlatina; only perception of light remained, pupils dilated. Bell. brought back the rash in three days and sight was restored in four weeks.—HUBBELL.

Amaurosis from a cold, with much vertigo, pressing pain and feeling of fulness in the eyeballs, black spots before the eyes, increased pain by candlelight and much congestion of the vessels. Cured by Bell.—LORBACHER.

Complete amaurosis caused by a severe nervous fever (?) or from the large amount of Quinine given at that time, pupils widely dilated. Cured.—FINDEISEN.

Amblyopia caused by stoppage of the menses, veil before the sight, diplopia, chromopsia, dilated pupils and stitching in the right eye. Cured.—HARTLAUB.

Blindness following severe congestive headaches after scarlet fever was restored. Triplopia, sees a second dim representation of the object on each side of it; from the candle proceed rays of the same color as the flame, and outside the rays there is a variegated halo, the inner circle being green, the middle red and the outer white; when walking he also sees a round black ball hovering, a little larger than a pea. All this he sees before his left eye. These symptoms disappeared under the influence of Bell.—BERRIDGE.

BORAX.

The lashes turn inward toward the eye and inflame it, especially in the outer canthus, where the margins of the lid are very sore. Flickering before the eyes in the morning when writing, so that he does not see distinctly; there seem to be bright moving waves, now from the right to the left side, now from above downward, several mornings in succession.

Clinical. Has been used in a few cases of trichiasis with benefit, but in the majority of cases is of no avail.

BOVISTA.

Clinical. A lady had for two years, "paralysis of the optic nerve" of right eye, with total blindness. When it first came on she could see just one-half of an object perpendicularly. Bovista^{200}, cured in four weeks.—BAKER.

BROMINE.

Clinical. According to Lippe, is most useful in fistula lachrymalis.

Should be borne in mind in the treatment of exophthalmic goitre.

BRYONIA.

Objective. Puffiness of the right upper lid. Morning agglutination and frequent lachrymation.

Subjective. Drawing together of the left upper lid, with a sensation of heaviness therein; aching pains in the eyes. Severe burning and lachrymation of the right eye. Very sensitive pressive pain (coming and going) in the left eyeball, *especially violent on moving the ball*, with a feeling as if the eye became smaller and retracted in the orbit.

Vision. Dim vision; on reading, the letters seem to run together; appearance of all the colors of the rainbow; every object seemed covered with these colors. Photophobia.

Clinical. It is found that Bryonia is rarely, if ever, indicated in diseases affecting the external tissues of the eye; its great sphere of usefulness being in diseases of the uveal tract.

Several cases of rheumatic iritis, caused from a cold, with a steady aching pain in the back part of the eye, extending through to the occiput, worse at night and on motion, have been cured. Is often indicated when the inflammation has extended to the choroid, as is shown in the following case of acute irido-choroiditis, in which opacities were present in the vitreous, iris tremulous, great ciliary injection, pus in the anterior chamber, eyeball sore on moving, and darting pains from the left eye through the head, with heaviness of the head afternoons. Bryonia speedily relieved.

In choroiditis uncomplicated with iritis, it is one of our chief remedies, especially in the *serous* or exudative forms, as one would be led to suppose from its relation to serous inflammations in general.

Glaucoma has occasionally been checked in its progress by Bryonia, if the eyeball feels full, as if pressed out, with sharp shooting pains in the eye and head, worse at night.

A case of hyperæmia of the optic nerve and retina, was immediately relieved by this drug; a bluish haze appeared before the vision, (vision $\frac{20}{50}$) with severe pain over the eye like a needle, going through the eyes and head, (compelling her to go to bed) with heat through the whole head, aggravated by stooping.

Ciliary neuralgia often requires Bryonia, especially if the pains are very sharp and severe, even making the patients scream out; the pains are aggravated by opening the eye and by any motion of the eyeball; the eyes must be kept closed and at rest. The pains, when this remedy is indicated, are usually *sharp in character, passing through the eye into the head or from the eye downward into malar region and thence backward to the occiput; the seat of pain becomes sore as a boil, and the least exertion, talking, moving or using the eyes, aggravates the trouble.*

The following symptoms have been reported as cured by this drug, though not found in any proving; some have been repeatedly verified and seem to direct the choice of the remedy. They are mostly variations of sensation in different persons, dependent upon the great characteristics of the remedy, aggravated by motion and ameliorated by pressure. Pressing, crushing pain in the eyes, worse on motion. Soreness and aching of the eyes upon moving them. Scalding in the corners of the eyes aggravated at night. Dull pain and soreness, especially in the left eye, worse in the morning and relieved by pressure.

CACTUS GRAND.

Clinical. From its action upon the heart, cases of exophthalmic goitre have been improved.

Angell advises its use in hyperæmia of the eye, especially of the fundus.

CALCAREA CARBONICA.

Objective. Swelling and redness of the lids with nightly agglutination; during the day they are full of mucus with a hot sensation, smarting pain and lachrymation. Lachrymation on writing.

Subjective. A painful sensation as if a foreign body were in the eye. Pressure and itching in the eyes; worse in the evening. Itching, burning, and stitches, especially on the margins of the lids and in the inner canthi.

Vision. Farsightedness. Only one side of objects visible, with dilated pupils. Dimness of the eyes after getting the head cold. Flickering, sparks and black spots before the eyes. Photophobia.

Clinical. The clinical record of this drug in superficial inflammations of the eye, is very full.

It has been found especially curative in various forms of blepharitis, occurring in unhealthy, "pot-bellied" children, inclined to grow fat, and who sweat profusely about the head; lids red, swollen and indurated; inflammation of the margins of the lids, causing loss of the eyelashes, with thick, purulent, excoriating discharge and burning, sticking pains; blepharitis with great itching in the lids.

Indurations remaining after styes and tarsal tumors have disappeared under its use.

Cases of entropion are reported cured.

Lachrymal fistulæ are on record as relieved.

The discharges from the eye are often profuse, and therefore this drug has been used with advantage in purulent ophthalmia, especially in that form found in new-born children, characterized by profuse yellowish white discharge, great swelling of the lids and ulceration of the cornea.

Conjunctivitis trachomatosa with pannus, much redness and lachrymation, caused from working in the wet, has been speedily relieved.

A marked illustration of the curative action of the drug in affections caused by working in water, is shown by the following case:—A boatman suffered for years from repeated attacks of sore eyes, caused by getting wet and cold. Pterygium developed and grew rapidly. Calc. c. speedily checked the progress of the disease, and when last seen, the cornea had cleared and but little thickness remained in the internal canthus.

Superficial keratitis or other forms of inflammation of the cornea, caused from getting wet or aggravated in damp weather, are quickly helped.

But it is particularly in scrofulous inflammations of the cornea and conjunctiva, as shown by pustules and ulcers, that Calc. c. proves so beneficial. The following case affords a good illustration of the prominent features of this drug. Keratitis pustulosa, with profuse lachrymation, excessive photophobia and sticking pains; lids closed, red and swollen, with painful itching in them; agglutination mornings; head scurfy; cervical glands swollen, also the upper lip; acrid discharge from the nose; eruptions that burn and itch; abdomen distended and hard; skin pale and flabby. After the administration of Calc. c., the above symptoms were promptly relieved and the eye restored. The photophobia and lachrymation are usually excessive, though we sometimes find cases, in which they are absent or only present in a moderate degree, though the general indications lead us to prescribe this remedy. The pains are more commonly sticking in character, though they may vary greatly. It is particularly applicable in inflammation of the eyes, occurring after the suppression of an eruption with mercury, if hardness of hearing is present at the same time.

Diffuse haziness of the cornea (interstitial keratitis) has been benefited.

Not only in inflammatory conditions of the cornea, but also in the sequelæ of such inflammations, as opacities of the cornea, has this remedy been serviceable.

Cases of squint, resulting from opacities of the cornea, are reported as relieved.

Asthenopia from hyperopia with pain in the eyes after using them, worse in damp weather and from warmth. The following symptoms found in asthenopia have also been verified. Burning and cutting pains in the lids, especially on reading, or sticking pains in the eyes with dull hearing. Dim vision after fine work, like a cloud before the eyes, objects run together with desire to close the eyes. Red and green halo around the light.

The selection of Calcarea will, in the majority of cases, depend mainly upon the general condition (cachexia) of the patient, since the eye symptoms are very often too general to individualize the remedy. The reverse may be said of Euphrasia and other remedies exhibiting no general dyscrasia.

CALCAREA CAUST.

Clinical. Has been recommended by Dr. Hills in granular lids, if the lids adhere in the morning and scurfs are found in the ciliæ during the day; especially when occurring in "chalky" scrofulous subjects; children during dentition or plethoric females with too early and profuse menstruation. Profuse perspiration about the neck and cold, clammy condition of the feet.

CALCAREA IODATA.

Clinical. The provings of this preparation of lime give us no clue to its sphere of action in diseases of the eye. But it is found by clinical observation to be an important remedy in scrofulous inflammations of the eyes and lids; as in chronic cases of blepharitis, complicated with enlargement of the tonsils.

It is, however, chiefly useful in pustules and ulcers, particularly of the cornea, marked by great photophobia, acrid lachrymation, sticking pains, and spasm of the lids; upon forcing open the lids, a stream of tears flow down the cheek; also erysipelatous swelling of the lids, chiefly of the upper, which is shining and red (compare Rhus). The inflammation of the eyes is always worse from the least cold, to which these cases are very susceptible. Is chiefly indicated in pale, fat subjects, who sweat much about the head, with enlargement of the tonsils and cervical glands. Only one eye is usually affected.

A case of kerato-conus (!) from superficial keratitis, with great photophobia, is reported by H. Goullon.

Decided benefit has been obtained from the use of the iodide of lime, in checking the progress of both conical cornea and staphyloma.

CALCAREA PHOSPHORICA.

Sensation as if something in the eyes; he always feels it anew, if even, after several days, it is only mentioned.

Cannot read; light hurts, particularly candle-light.

Clinical. A case of keratitis occurring in a girl, æt. 16, after small-pox, was cured by Calc. phos.:—Left eye much inflamed, cornea hazy, particularly the upper portion and traversed by red vessels, photophobia.—R. T. Cooper.

CALENDULA.

Clinical. Calendula has been employed with great success in injuries of the eye and its appendages. It is especially applicable to cut-wounds.

In wounds of lids and brows which have been badly treated by plasters, etc., until suppuration has taken place, the local application of Calendula is the remedy.

After all operations upon the eye or lids, this drug is useful in preventing any undue amount of inflammation and in hastening recovery.

Blennorrhœa of the lachrymal sac has been benefited.

In traumatic conjunctivitis, keratitis and iritis it has proved of service.

It has only occasionally been used internally, being usually applied locally, in the proportion of ten drops of the tincture to the ounce of water or even stronger. Probably a better preparation for the eye is a decoction, made from the leaves.

CANNABIS SATIVA.

The cornea becomes obscured (film before the eyes).

Sensation of spasmodic drawing in the eye; as if sand were in the eyes. Pressure from behind the eye forwards.

Clinical. From its clinical record, this drug seems to be especially adapted to non-inflammatory conditions of the cornea, or to that form of inflammation marked by no active inflammatory symptoms. For instance, several cases of opacities of the cornea have been reported cured, particularly when occurring without any previous active inflammation.

In keratitis parenchymatosa (not pannus), in which the whole thickness of the cornea is red and vascular, it is said to have been found useful, though this is the only form of inflammation of the eye (and this is very chronic in nature) in which our literature shows Cannabis to have been used with benefit.

Cataract is reported to have been cured by this remedy, but it seems a matter of considerable doubt.

CANTHARIS.

Eyes red and suffused with tears; margins of lids sore and painful. Burning in the eyes and glowing heat, as from coals. Biting sensation, as if salt were in them.

Clinical. Has been used with benefit in inflammations of the eye, caused from a burn, as in the case of a young man who had had a hot iron thrust into the eye, burning the conjunctiva and thus producing quite a severe conjunctivitis, with burning pain in the eye. Canth. quickly relieved the pain and cured.

CARBO VEGETABILIS.

Subjective. A heavy weight seemed to be upon the eyes, so that he must make a great exertion when reading or writing, in order to distinguish letters. The muscles of the eye pain when looking up. Itching in the margin of the lids and about the eyes.

Vision. He became short-sighted after exerting the eyes for some time. Black floating spots, flickering and rings before the eyes.

Clinical. This drug has been too little employed in eye-diseases and its clinical history is extremely scant.

In asthenopia, as the verified symptoms indicate, it has proved beneficial.

From its symptomatology we are led to recommend its use in cases of myopia, accompanied by posterior staphyloma, in which it ought to relieve the unpleasant symptoms and prevent the increase of the staphyloma, though we do not imagine that it would in any degree diminish the amount of myopia.

CARBOLIC ACID.

Very severe supra-orbital neuralgia over the right eye. Slight pain over the right eyeball; the same kind of pain, but in a milder degree, under right patella, both of short duration.

While writing, the letters seem to run together. A constant dark spot in front of the left eye.

Clinical. This remedy having been of only comparatively recent addition to our Materia Medica, has been very little employed in diseases of the eye, though it has proved very useful in some cases of supra-orbital neuralgia, as indicated by the symptoms given above.

CAUSTICUM.

Objective. Inflammation of the eyes, with burning and pressure in them and agglutination in the morning. Visible twitching of the lids and in the left eyebrow Lachrymation even in a warm room, but worse in the open air.

Subjective. Burning and stinging as with needles in the eyes, with dryness and photophobia, especially in the evening. Pressure in the eyes as if sand were in them. Pressive pain in the eye increased by touch. Biting and pressure in the eyes, which seem heavy, with redness of the lid. Itching of the eyes, especially in the lids; disappears on rubbing. Inclination to close the eyes; they close involuntarily. *Sensation of heaviness in the upper lid, as if he could not raise it easily* or as if it were agglutinated to the lower lid and could not be easily loosened. Opening of the lids is difficult. Itching on the lower lid and on its inner surface, with burning as soon as he touches the eye or moves it.

Vision. Photophobia; constantly obliged to wink. Flickering before the eyes, as from swarms of insects. If he winks, he sees sparks of fire before the eyes, even on a bright day. The eyes become dim, and the vision indistinct; it seems as though a thick cloud were before the eyes. Obscuration of the vision, as if a veil were drawn before them; transient obscuration on blowing the nose.

Clinical. From the symptomatology given above and the many verifications, it will be readily seen how important a remedy this must be in ophthalmic diseases.

In affections of the lids it has proved very useful, as in some cases of blepharitis, (especially if ameliorated in the fresh air—Liebold), also in certain forms of tumors of the lids, particularly warts found on the lids and brows.

In scrofulous inflammations of the eye it has been used with great benefit, as in inflammation of the eyes, with corrosive lachrymation and shooting pains, extending up into the head, worse in the evening and at night, with a green halo around the light; in chronic inflammation of the eyes with violent shooting pains, dimness of vision and noises in the head; inflammation with smarting in the eyes, as if worried or irritated without much lachrymation; also scrofulous inflammation of the eyes, in which the cornea is covered by red vessels and has a tendency to bulge.

Cases of trachoma with pannus have been greatly helped.

The action of Caust. upon the lens is probably as pronounced as any remedy in our materia medica, and several cases of cataract have been arrested in their progress and the sight even improved, where, before its administration, they were rapidly going on to complete blindness. The following case will illustrate its action:—A man appeared for treatment with well marked hard cataract, which was rapidly increasing. (Had been told by celebrated oculists of the old school that he would soon be blind and that he then could be operated upon.) He complained of the following symptoms, a sensation as if there was a substance in the eye too large, causing a kind of heaviness and distension only in the evening, also a feeling as if there was something moving in the eyes in the evening; cannot retain his urine, and could not feel the urine passing through the urethra. Under the influence of Caust. the progress of the cataract was immediately checked, and one year afterwards the vision was found somewhat improved, though the white striæ in the lens underwent no appreciable change. After seven years his vision remains fully as good as when he began treatment.

But its principal sphere of action is in paralysis of the muscles, and here it is the remedy "par excellence." It has been used more often with advantage in paralysis of the external rectus, levator palpebræ superioris and orbicularis, though indicated in paralysis of any of the muscles, particularly if caused from exposure to cold. Partial paralysis of the orbicularis with great lachrymation, are known to have been cured, as well as many cases of ptosis caused by cold.

A lady, thirty-two, after being heated by dancing, took cold and was taken in the night with severe tearing pains in the left half of the face; afterward she saw indistinctly; diplopia followed with inability to turn the left eye outward (paresis N. abducentis sin). Caust. removed the paresis entirely in fourteen days.—PAYR.

Paralysis of the muscles resulting from exposure to wet, more generally calls for Rhus than for Caust.

CEDRON.

Pain across the eyes from temple to temple. *Severe shooting pain over the left eye.*

Clinical. The sphere of usefulness of Cedron, so far as experience has taught us, is confined to neuralgic affections of the eye, particularly when involving the supra-orbital nerve; and in supra-orbital neuralgia it is among the first remedies to be thought of. The pains are usually severe, sharp and shooting, starting from one point over the eye, (more often over the left) and then extending along the branches of the supra-orbital nerve up into the head; in some cases the pains have been worse in the evening and upon lying down, though this may not be characteristic. One case of pressing frontal headache of long standing, occurring in a woman troubled with chronic disseminate choroiditis, with sharp pains extending from above the eyes back to the temples and occiput, and always worse before a storm, was very quickly and permanently relieved by a few doses of Cedron^3.

The severe supra-orbital pains found in iritis, choroiditis and other deep inflammations of the eye, are often speedily controlled by this drug.

CHAMOMILLA.

Objective. The eyelids are swollen in the morning and agglutinated with purulent mucus; much discharge of pus or blood. Conjunctiva swollen and dark red. Lachrymation.

Subjective. Burning and sensation of heat in the eyes; pressure in the eyes, which are inflamed and full of mucus in the morning. Violent pressure in the orbital region, sensation in the eyeball as if it were compressed from all sides, with momentary obscuration of vision. Stitches in the orbital region and soreness in the canthi.

Clinical. Is especially adapted to superficial inflammations of the eye, occurring in children, being rarely, if ever, useful in diseases of the deeper tissues.

According to Tülf, has been employed with benefit in blepharo-adenitis catarrhalis, with no lachrymation; lids painful on opening and closing, and agglutinated mornings.

Is an excellent remedy in ophthalmia neonatorum, characterized by the usual symptoms, (even if the cornea has been attacked) if the child is very fretful and wants to be carried all the time; also in inflammation of the conjunctiva in children, if that tissue is so much congested that blood oozes out drop by drop from between the swollen lids (Nux), especially marked upon any attempt to open them.

Cham. has proven very serviceable in many cases of scrofulous ophthalmia occurring in cross peevish children during dentition, and it will often relieve the severity of the symptoms, even though it does not complete the cure. The symptoms which call for this drug are usually severe; the pustules and ulcers are chiefly situated on the cornea, and are attended with great intolerance to light, considerable redness and lachrymation.

CHELIDONIUM MAJUS.

Objective. Twitching and blinking of the lids. The white of the eye is of a dirty-yellow color. Lachrymation.

Subjective. Tearing pain in and above the eyes. Neuralgic pain above the right eye, especially in the evening when reading by artificial light. Pressive pain above the left eye, which seems to press down the upper lid. Aching in the eyeballs on looking up or moving the eyes.

Vision. Dimness of vision. A blinding spot seems to be before the eyes, and if he looks at it, the eye waters.

Clinical. At one time this drug was employed in a variety of eye troubles, and with some success, but of late it seems to have fallen into disuse.

Buchmann reports a case of severe inflammation of the eye cured by Chel.[6], occurring in a man, æt. 62, caused by getting the feet wet; lids thick, red, swollen and lashes partially absent; conjunctiva swollen and dark red; thick yellow discharge from the eyes, agglutination mornings, and great photophobia, with burning, sticking pains in the eyes.

Maculæ corneæ and even cataract are reported cured by material doses of this drug, but this has failed of later verifications.

In A. H. Z., Firmat gives a description of five cases of intermittent ciliary neuralgia, in which Chel. gave immediate relief. The cases were all very similar to each other and were marked by the following symptoms:—The attacks appeared every day, usually early in the morning or forenoon, and were ushered in by yawning and shivering, which would be soon followed by beating, pulsating, burning or sticking pain over the eyes (usually over one eye, the right), which would steadily increase until it became almost unbearable, extending up into the forehead and temples and down into the eye, which would become red, sensitive to light and watery; the eye would become painful, as if pressed together from before backward in some cases, while in others would be more of a tearing sensation; pressure with the hand would relieve the pain momentarily; but any movement, exposure to light or open air, would aggravate. The attacks would terminate in the afternoon on the breaking out of a light sweat. The second or third potency was usually employed.*

* We have failed to observe good effects from Chel. in similar cases.

Amaurosis resulting from rheumatic troubles, and amaurosis brought on from the suppression of a ringworm by red precipitate ointment, are on record as cured.

CHIMAPHILA UMBELLATA.

Clinical. A large number of cases of pterygium have been treated by this drug, a few of which have shown marked improvement, while others have exhibited no good results from its use.

CHINA.

Motion of eyes painful, with sensation of mechanical hindrance. Lachrymation, with crawling pains in the eyes and in the inner surface of the lids. Dimness of vision.

Clinical. Has been successfully employed in a variety of eye troubles, but is especially indicated in those diseases of a malarial origin and intermittent character; also in those affections in which there is impairment of tone from loss of vital fluids.

A case of scrofulous ophthalmia marked by a pressing pain in one spot at the inner and upper border of the orbit, extending to the nose and sometimes into the lid, closing it, and of an intermittent type, coming on every evening about eleven o'clock, was cured by China.—Caspari.

In ulceration of the cornea, dependent upon malarial causes or anæmic conditions, especially when the iris becomes complicated (kerato-iritis), we have here an excellent remedy.

Is useful in some cases of iritis if caused from the loss of vital fluids, as in one case reported by Arnold, in which it came on from the loss of blood after confinement. Again it cured a very severe attack of iritis (probably kerato-iritis) in the right eye, from inoculation with gonorrhœal virus, in which the photophobia was intense, even extending to the other eye with severe constant pain in the forehead.

In intermittent ciliary neuralgia it has proved very beneficial, when there was painful pressure and drawing in the forehead and temples every day at 10 A.M., lasting some three hours; general excitation during the attack and depression after; every touch or motion aggravates the pain.—RAUE.

Also when the pain has been excessive as if a knife were thrust between the orbit and ball, and moved about in the orbital cavity as if to scoop out the eye, commencing at 8 A.M. and continuing till 2 or 3 P.M.—ST. MARTIN.

Quinine has cured some cases of neuritis.

Hemeralopia, with no other abnormal symptoms, is on record as cured.

Has been used with benefit in several forms of amblyopia, especially if due to venereal excesses, masturbation or loss of any fluids. A case of amblyopia consequent upon venereal excesses and intoxication, is reported, in which large objects could be distinguished at six paces; letters run together and look pale like black spots on a white ground; pupils dilated and sluggish; fundus of the eye hazy, cornea dim; vision better in the morning; associated with loss of strength, trembling of the hands, weak digestion and uneasy sleep. Within four weeks after the use of China 1st and 2d, was able to read usual print. —CASPARI.

Dr. Steus also reports a case of "amaurosis" associated with spinal irritation; she suddenly became blind in the right eye and soon after in the left. In this case most violent pain in the occiput extending over the head into the eyes, with great sensitiveness of the spine and swollen spleen were the characteristic symptoms present. China[1] produced first an aggravation, followed by a sudden return of vision, first in the left eye, afterward in the right.

CHININUM MURIATICUM.

Clinical. This form of Quinine, in appreciable doses, has been used with great success in controlling the severe neuralgic pains occurring in iritis and various other diseases of the eye.

Is often called for in ulceration of the cornea, if the iris has become affected and we have *severe pain*, either in the eye or above, *periodic in character*, especially if accompanied by chills; also in ulcers complicating pannus, with much pain in the morning. The intensity of the pains and their intermittent character will furnish our chief indications.

The attention of some of the surgeons of the N. Y. Ophthalmic Hospital was called to this drug by Dr. Belcher, since which the above observations have been repeatedly verified.

Very favorable results have been observed from its use in trachoma, with and without pannus.

CHININUM SULPHURICUM.

Eyes lustreless and restless. Disk and retina both very anæmic. Pupils dilated. Neuralgic twinges in the supra and infra-orbital nerves, generally periodic in character.

Vision. Dimness of vision as from a net before the eyes, and as from a dark fog. Great sensitiveness of the eye to the light, with lachrymation in the full glare of light. Bright light and sparks before the eyes. Black spot size of pin's head, about eighteen inches from right eye and moving with eye for some weeks.

Clinical. An interesting case of intermittent strabismus occurring in a child and continuing for some time, would squint one day and be entirely well on the next, was cured by the use of this remedy in the hands of an empiric.

Herschman reports the following case which came on after bathing:—The conjunctiva was injected, lids red and swollen, pupils contracted, lachrymation, extreme photophobia, tearing heat in the orbit and headache, with thirst and fever; all appearing every second day. Chin. sulph. cured.

Can only see objects when looking at them sideways. Chin. sulph.^{200}, one dose relieved.—BERRIDGE.

CHLORAL.

Clinical. A number of cases of "ophthalmia" have been relieved and cured by this drug. One grain of the pure salts dissolved in water, three times a day for adults, and a fraction of a grain for children.—D. DYCE BROWN.

CICUTA VIROSA.

Objective. Eyes staring; she stares with unaltered look at one and the same place, and cannot help it. Pupils dilated and insensible. Pupils first contracted then dilated.

Vision. When she attempts to stand, she wishes to hold on to something, because objects seem now to come nearer, and now to recede from her. Objects seem double (and black).

Clinical. It is in spasmodic affections of the eye and its appendages, that this remedy is especially indicated; thus we find it very valuable in strabismus, particularly if periodic and of a spasmodic character; many cases of which have been cured, (this, of course, excludes that form of periodic squint dependent upon an anomaly of refraction). Strabismus occurring after a fall or blow, has been relieved.

A case reported by ———, shows that it is useful in spasmodic action of other muscles besides the recti, viz.:—Trembling and twitching of the lids, extending even to the face, of six months standing, was cured in fifteen hours by Cicuta[15].

Caspari narrates the following symptoms found in a patient which Cicuta relieved:—Letters seem to be twisted, and they, as well as a light, have a rainbow appearance around them; upon attempting to use the eyes she becomes dizzy and objects appear to waver; there is also photophobia, sometimes burning in the eyes, dilated pupils, morning agglutination, blue borders around the eyes and headache over the eyes.

CIMICIFUGA.

Eyes congested during headache. Pain over the eyes, extending from them to the top of the head. Pain in the centre of the eyeballs, and also sensation as if pain were situated between the eyeball and the orbital plate of the parietal bone, worse in the morning. *Aching pain in both eyeballs.* Black specks before the eyes.

Clinical. This is not a remedy often called for if there has been much tissue change, unless it be to control the pains which arise in the course of the disease.

Ulceration of the cornea has, however, in a few instances been cured, if accompanied by sharp pains through the eye into the head.

In certain forms of ciliary neuralgia its value has been often proven. It is indicated by *aching pains* in the eyeball or in the temples, extending to the eyes, so severe, especially at night, in some instances that it seemed as if the patient would go crazy; also if the pains are of a sharp shooting character, going from the occiput through to the eyes, or especially if they seem to dart from the eyes up to the top of the head; these pains often produce some redness of the eye, photophobia, etc., and are generally worse on the right side, in the afternoon and at night, and ameliorated on lying down.

Macrotin has been employed in a variety of ophthalmic disorders, but like Cimicifuga, is particularly adapted to ciliary neuralgia, as the following case reported by F. B. Sherburne, will illustrate:—Frank B., æt. 20, was attacked with a slight pain in the back part of the orbit, near the foramen, with photophobia. The ophthalmoscope reveals no interior change. Photophobia, pain in temples, soreness in back part of eyeballs have steadily increased. Movement produces very severe pain as though the globes would be torn from the orbits. Treatment consisted of Macrot., two drops per dose, every two hours, which cured the patient even while attending to his daily duties.

CINA.

Pulsation of the superciliary muscles; a kind of convulsion. A slow stitch extending from above the upper orbital margin deep into the brain. Pupils dilated.

On rising from the bed it becomes black before the eyes, with dizziness in the head and faintness; he totters to and fro; relieved on lying down.

Clinical. Cina has been strongly recommended and often used with benefit in strabismus, dependent upon helminthiasis, if the child has a pale sickly look, blue rings around the eyes, pains about the umbilicus, frequent urination, boring of the nose, etc.

Chronic weakness of the eyes, with aching in them and photophobia, as the result of onanism has been removed.

Santonine has been successfully employed, especially in asthenopia, and also in a case of amaurosis, as follows:—Asthenopia. A young lady at school complains that while studying, the sight becomes suddenly dim and the letters indistinct; while reading fast, the same symptoms are aggravated; rubbing the eyes seem to clear up the vision. Santonine, 2d dec., three doses per day for two weeks, removed the trouble.—W. R. McLaren.

When the exciting cause of asthenopia is some refractive anomaly, Santonine, 2d dec., night and morning, will often produce a favorable result.—Woodyatt.

Bærtl reports a case of complete amaurosis coming on suddenly, in a soldier, with slight dilatation of the pupil; helminthiasis was supposed to be the cause. Under the administration of Santonine, six grains, three times daily, recovery took place.

CINNABARIS.

Pain from the inner canthus of left eye across the eyebrows.

Clinical. This form of Mercury is an important remedy in ophthalmic troubles, and the indications for its use are usually very clear.

4

In various forms of blepharitis, conjunctivitis and keratitis, even when severe ulceration of the cornea has occurred, it has proved especially serviceable if accompanied by that characteristic symptom of *pain above the eye, extending from the internal to the external canthus, or a pain which runs around the eye, usually above but sometimes below;* this pain may vary greatly in intensity or character, being sometimes sharp, stinging or stitching, at other times dull or aching, and may extend into the eye or up into the head. The photophobia and lachrymation are usually very marked, as well as the redness. The lids frequently feel so heavy that it is with difficulty they are kept open, especially in the evening.

In kerato-iritis and in uncomplicated iritis it is often called for, especially in the syphilitic variety and if condylomata are present on the iris, and even on the lids. Our chief indication will be found in the characteristic pain already given, though there is often present besides, shooting pains through the eye into the head, soreness along the course of the supra-orbital nerve and corresponding side of the head, with nocturnal aggravation.

Asthenopia, with pain extending from inner canthus around the eye, with soreness over the exit of the supra-orbital nerve, worse in the morning, has been relieved.

Should always be thought of in ciliary neuralgia, in which it has proved a very valuable remedy, as might be expected from the character of the pains already mentioned.

CLEMATIS.

Clinical. Has been found of value in chronic, irritable conditions of the lids, with swelling of the meibomian glands, occurring in young scrofulous subjects; also in pustular conjunctivitis complicated with tinea capitis, lids agglutinated in the morning.

It is, however, in iritis and kerato-iritis, that most benefit has been derived from Clematis (and by some it is considered equal to mercury); in these cases there is usually much dryness and burning heat in the eyes, as if fire were streaming from them, great *sensitiveness to cold air*, to light or bathing; in many respects the symptoms are similar to Merc.

Posterior Synechiæ are said to have been helped.

COCCULUS.

Bruised pain in the eyes, with inability to open the lids at night. Dimness of vision.

Clinical. Upon record are to be found two cases of "arthritic ophthalmia" in which this drug effected a cure (Thorer). One of these was undoubtedly a case of glaucoma in a rheumatic subject, marked by venous hyperæmia, dilated pupils, insensibility to light, haziness of the lens and vitreous, most severe, tearing pain in and around the eyes, etc.; the other seems to have been iritis, with corneal and scleral complication, especially affecting the left eye, in which the iris was inflamed as well as the sclera, pupil irregular and contracted, blue border around the cornea, which was dim, photophobia, no lachrymation, and tearing pains in the brow and left side of the head, worse in the evening and at night. Cocc.[12] was administered in both cases.

Kallenbach also recommends its use in similar cases.

COLCHICUM.

Clinical. Ulceration of the meibomian glands of the left lower lid, which is much swollen, and accompanied by great nervousness; also styes on the left lower lid near the inner canthus have been cured.

Painful tearing, drawing pains in the left side of the head, from the eye to the occiput, have been relieved.

(In a case of poisoning by Colchicum, severe hypopion was produced, therefore we might think of its use in this trouble.)

COLOCYNTHIS.

Painful pressure in the eyeballs, especially on stooping. Pain in the eyes; a sharp cutting in the right eyeball.

Clinical. Chiefly serviceable in controlling the pains of iritis and glaucoma, which are severe, burning, sticking and cutting, extending from the eye up into the head and around the eye, or else an aching pain going back into the head, usually worse on rest at night and on stooping, and *ameliorated by firm pressure* and walking in a warm room; a sensation on stooping as if the eye would fall out, is also sometimes present. The lachrymation is profuse (and acrid).

COMOCLADIA.

The eyes feel very heavy, larger than usual, painful and pressing out of the head, as if something was pressing on the top of the eyeballs, moving them downward and outward. Right eye very painful, feeling much larger and more protruded than the left. The eyes feel more painful when near the warm stove. Right eyeball very sore, worse on moving the eye. Eyeballs feel worse on moving them.

Clinical. Ciliary neuralgia from asthenopia and from chronic iritis have been relieved when indicated by the above symptoms.

CONIUM MACULATUM.

Objective. Whites of the eye yellow. Affected with a weakness and dazzling of the eyes, together with a giddiness and debility of the whole body, especially the muscles of the arms and legs, so that on attempting to walk one staggers like a person who had drunk too much liquor. Partially paralyzed condition of the external muscles of the eye; he could hardly raise the eyelids, which seemed pressed down by a heavy weight, and was disposed to fall off to sleep. Pupils dilated.

Subjective. Burning in the eyes and on the inner surface of the lids.

Vision. Double vision. Sluggishness of accommodation; vision good for fixed objects, but when an object is put in motion before eyes, there is a haze and dimness of vision, producing vertigo.

Clinical. In superficial inflammations of the eye we have in Conium a remedy of the first importance, but when the deeper structures become invaded, not as much benefit has, as yet, been obtained from its use.

Indurations of the lids have been removed, and ptosis has been benefited by Conium.

Two cases of blennorrhœa of the lachrymal sac are reported by Kirsten cured.

It is, however, in inflammatory conditions of the cornea (ulcers and pustules) that this remedy is chiefly useful, especially if the inflammation is superficial, involving only the epithelial layers, and whether caused from an injury, cold or scrofulous diathesis; the latter of which is most frequently the case. The indications for its use are generally very clear and well marked; thus, the *photophobia*, which is the most prominent symptom, *is excessive*, so that it is with great difficulty that we are enabled to open the spasmodically closed lids, and when they are opened, a profuse flow of hot tears take place (Rhus). Upon examination of the eye we usually find *very slight or no redness*, not sufficient to account for the great photophobia, which is out of all proportion to the amount of trouble. The discharge of mucus or pus is rarely profuse, but intimately mixed with the tears. The pains vary greatly, but are generally worse at night (eye aches on lying down to sleep) and in any light, relieved in a dark room and sometimes by pressure. Hence it appears that Conium is chiefly adapted to those cases, in which the nerves are in a state of hyperæsthesia, or when only the terminal filaments are exposed by superficial abrasion of the epithelial layer.

Keratitis punctata, accompanied by great photophobia, has been greatly benefited by this drug.

Kirsch reports a case of gray cataract, occurring in the left eye, the right having already been operated, which was cured with Conium^{200} (!).

Its use in hyperæsthesia of the retina should be borne in mind, as it has proved useful in this disorder.

By reference to its symptomatology, it will be seen that it must be important in paralysis of the muscles.

The following case, rapidly cured with Conium, illustrates its use in asthenopia:—Can read only a few seconds before the letters run together; burning pain deep in the eyes, with hot flashes; cannot bear either light or heat, is worse in a warm room, and better in the mornings and on a cloudy day; black spots are seen on closing the eyes; distant objects appear more distant; objects are surrounded by prismatic colors, out-of-doors; eyes perfectly normal in appearance.

The following symptoms found in a case reported by R. T. Cooper, were relieved by Conium^{30}. Eyes feel as if pulled outwards from the nose (external rectus muscle); photophobia; vertical pain in head, worse in the open air; often has to leave school from a sensation of overpowering giddiness coming over her; far-sighted.

CROCUS SATIVUS.

Objective. Visible twitching of the lids, with a sensation as if something must be wiped from the right eye. Inclined to press the eyes tightly together from time to time. Pupils dilated.

Subjective. Feeling in the eyes as though he had wept very violently. After reading a while (even during the day) the eyes pain, with a sore burning and some dimness, so that he was frequently obliged to wink. Feeling as of biting smoke in the eyes. Feeling as though water were constantly coming into the eyes, only in the room, not in the open air.

Vision. The light seems dimmer than usual, as if a veil were between the eyes and the light; is frequently obliged to wink and to wipe his eyes, as though a film of mucus were over them.

Clinical. This remedy has been but little employed in ophthalmic disorders, though Tülf remarks that "it is especially useful in ophthalmia menstrualis, occurring in patients of a sanguine temperament, who are subject to attacks of congestion and inclination to spasms (hysterical) at the climacteric; pressive pains and heaviness of the lids as if forced together, with sensation of dryness in the eyes; burning and itching in the lids; twitching of the lids, with a feeling as if something were in the eye to be washed away; great irritability of the eye and severe lachrymation on the slightest exertion of the eye; pupil either contracted or dilated; aggravation in the evening or in a warm room and amelioration in the open air."

The following symptoms found in a patient suffering from sclero-choroiditis post., were quickly removed by this drug:—Pain in the eye to the top of the head (Cimicif., Lach.), pain in the left eye darting to the right; also a sensation of cold wind blowing across the eyes (Fluoric acid).

Marked improvement has been observed from its use in asthenopia when indicated by symptoms given above.

Constant winking, with suffusion of the eyes in tears, found in a woman, was speedily relieved by Crocus^{200}.—J. T. O'CONNOR.

A feeling in the eyes as from violent weeping, especially if complicated with the sensation as if something were alive in the abdomen, is well marked and has been relieved by Crocus.

CROTALUS HORRIDUS.

Yellow color of the eyes. Blood exudes from the eye. Pressure and oppression above the eyes.

Clinical. Nunez advises the use of this remedy for clearing up the vision after an attack of keratitis or kerato-iritis.

Décran used it with benefit in a case of ciliary neuralgia in a woman, 25 years of age, who for two months had complained of tearing, boring pain, as if a cut had been made around the eye, sometimes sticking in character and worse morning and evening; great sensitiveness to light, especially lamp-light; lids swollen in the morning, with pains in the forehead and occiput; palpitation of heart, especially at menstrual periods. Also in another case of amblyopia, caused from grief and over-use of the eyes in sewing; cutting pains around the eyes were present, as well as muscæ volitantes and various colored flames before the vision.

Another great use for Crotalus, in common with the other snake poisons, as suggested by Dr. Liebold, is to be found in hemorrhages into the retina, whether occurring during the course of retinitis albuminurica and other diseases, or when it seems to be of spontaneous origin. It has not, as yet, been used as extensively as Lachesis in this condition, though it, no doubt, has similar properties.

CROTON TIGLIUM.

Irritation and inflammatory redness of the conjunctiva. Violent ophthalmia; on the second day, ulceration of the conjunctiva over the cornea and sclera, irritation of the sclera and iris; contraction of the pupil; injected state of the vessels of the conjunctiva, sclera and eyelids, profuse lachrymation, photophobia, violent pains disturbing the night's rest. Burning and violent pain of the eye.

Clinical. In Crot. tig. we have a valuable remedy for superficial inflammations of the eye, especially of the pustular variety.

Pustular eruptions found upon the lids either with or without any corneal or conjunctival complication, especially call for the use of this remedy and are quickly removed by it. Unless this appearance is present, is rarely indicated in blepharitis.

In phlyctenular keratitis and conjunctivitis its chief sphere of action is found. There is usually complicated with this condition a corresponding characteristic eruption on the face and lids; the eyes and face feel hot and burning, the photophobia is marked, ciliary injection like iritis, with considerable pain in and around the eye, usually worse at night.

It is not, however, confined to pustular inflammation in its first stage, but is useful when the pustules have terminated in ulcers and also in real ulceration of the cornea, especially if there is much pain in the supra-ciliary region and an eruption on the face. In one case there was always much pain in the eye, whenever a movement from the bowels occurred. Crot. tig. immediately relieved.

In iritis it is valuable, and claims our attention whenever accompanied by pustular eruption of the face.

CUPRUM ACETICUM.

Clinical. This preparation of copper has not been extensively employed in diseases of the eye, though an interesting case of paralysis of the nervus abducentis of the left eye is reported by C. Heingke in H. Kl. A young man, æt. 29, was suddenly taken on leaving the cars, after several hours of railroad ride, with indistinct and double vision. The above diagnosis was fully confirmed, and electricity with iodide of potash was used for three months with no change. No other symptoms were present, with the exception of slight frontal headache of which the patient had been suffering for years. Sulph. and Rhus did little good. Cuprum acet., first 3, then 6 and afterward 30, in repeated doses and at gradually increasing intervals, cured the case within a few months.

CUPRUM ALUMINATUM.

Clinical. The aluminate of copper has been successfully used to a great extent in trachoma, to which condition it seems especially adapted. The results obtained are usually more satisfactory than those found from the sulphate of copper, which is the main reliance of the old school in the treatment of this disorder. It is used locally by application of the crystals to the granulations, at the same time giving the remedy in the potencies internally.

Battmann relates five cases of ophthalmia neonatorum, characterized by all the usual symptoms in which other remedies had failed; and Cuprum al., one grain to the ounce of water, two or three drops of which instilled into the eye, from four to six times a day, effected rapid cures. He has also used the same solution with satisfactory results in chronic catarrhal ophthalmia, especially if there be morning agglutination.

Conjunctivitis pustulosa with inflammation of the lids, has been cured by the administration of this drug.

Great benefit has also been derived from its application to opacities of the cornea.

CUPRUM SULPHURICUM.

Clinical. Is considered by the old school, one of their most efficient remedies for many superficial troubles of the eye; chief among which may be mentioned granular lids.

Has also proved beneficial in both catarrhal and purulent conjunctivitis, if used locally.

CYCLAMEN.

Clinical. Very little use has been made of this drug in ophthalmic diseases, still, from what is known, it must rank among our most important remedial agents for convergent strabismus. Eidherr and others have reported cases cured. Various forms of diplopia are said to have been relieved, especially if dependent upon convergent squint, arising from helminthiasis, convulsions, falls, etc.

A woman, æt. 30, was nearly blind (amblyopia); came on

after the suppression of an eruption; she has never menstruated, though has much headache and vertigo at the time the menses ought to appear. Cyclamen brought on the menstrual flow and restored the vision.—Eidherr.

Hemiopia, only the left half of the object is visible, is said to have been relieved.

DIGITALIS.

Meibomian glands inflamed. Lachrymation, worse in a room; eyes are dim, hot, congested, with pressive pain; mucus in canthi.

Objects seem green or yellow. Hemiopia, as if the upper part of the field of vision were covered by a dark cloud evenings while walking. (Digitalin).

Clinical. Has proved useful in some cases of superficial inflammation of the eye and its appendages, as in blepharoadenitis; also in a case of catarrhal inflammation of the eye occurring after the disappearance of a coryza, conjunctiva red, lids swollen, great photophobia, constant lachrymation, worse in the light or cold air, copious secretion of purulent mucus accumulating in the canthi during the night, burning in the eyes, feeling of sand in them and stitches darting through, with stoppage and dryness of the nose.—Knorre.

Benefit has also been obtained from Dig. in checking the progress of detachment of the retina and in relieving some of the troublesome symptoms, as wavering, everything appears green or yellow, etc.

DULCAMARA.

Clinical. Dr. Wesselhœft has cured several cases of ophthalmia neonatorum (often accompanied by constipation), with chemosis of the conjunctiva.

ELAPS CORALLINUS.

Clinical. A man, 61 years of age, had been completely blind in the left eye for three years, and nearly so in the right for three months, following headache. Now has severe headache with drawing, sometimes sticking pains from the forehead to the occiput; pain at the root of the nose with vertigo. Even with the right eye he can scarcely tell light from dark; *everything seems white*, even at night. Some old rheumatic symptoms in the hips. Was cured by the lower preparations of Elaps.—DÉCRAN.

ELECTRICITY AND GALVANISM.

Clinical. A man, æt. 27, troubled with granular ophthalmia, had tried everything till nearly blind. Electricity, fifteen minutes daily, cured in nine weeks.—A. H. O., 6, 145.

Galvanism is reported to have removed cataract and leucoma.—LERCHE. Also to have cured rheumatic ophthalmia.—HALLE.

Posterior synechiæ are said to give way under the influence of a current of electricity passed through the eye; and opacities of the vitreous have also been absorbed by the same means.

The use of the magnet is reported to have relieved the intense photophobia found in scrofulous ophthalmia.

A case of amblyopia in a man 45 years old:—Appears as if a dark cloud covered everything; better after eating, was cured by electricity.—HILBERGER.

It is, however, in paralysis of the muscles and weakness of the internal recti (asthenopia muscularis) that electricity proves itself chiefly serviceable.

Cases of paralysis both complete and partial of all the ocular muscles, have been restored by the aid of electricity or galvanism, though usually some remedy has been employed at the same time internally, as Caust., Rhus, Euphras., etc. It is usually applied by placing one pole (some say the positive and others the negative) over the affected muscle, while the other is passed lightly over the corresponding brow or in some cases placed at the back of the neck; it should be applied regularly every day or two, for about three minutes at one sitting.*

EUPATORIUM PERFOLIATUM.

Clinical. Soreness of the eyeballs; intolerance to light; redness of the margins of the lids, with glutinous secretion from the meibomian glands and increased lachrymation, are symptoms which have been verified.

EUPHORBIUM.

Clinical. Of benefit in chronic ophthalmia if the lids pain and itch severely, are wet and agglutinated.

Cataract in a man aged 55:—Lens milk white; cannot see to go alone, though sees better in a dark day. Large development of abdominal organs, but otherwise seemed to be perfectly healthy. Euphorb. tinct. cured him so that he was able to read.—Bojanus.

EUPHRASIA.

Objective. Lids red and swollen, at times an itching burning, with increased watery discharge. Swelling of ciliary margin of lids with dry sensation. Lids partly closed. Eyes sore and discharge almost to blinding.

Lachrymation profuse; tears acrid and burning. Coryza mild and bland, with burning tears. *Catarrhal inflammation of the eyes and nasal organs, with profuse secretion of acrid mucus* from

* Much use is now being made of reversed currents by most eminent electricians.

the eyes and nose, with pain in the frontal sinuses. Conjunctiva chemosed.

Subjective. Aching in the eyes, must wink frequently. Sense as if cornea were covered by mucus, it blinds him and forces one to frequently close and press the eyes together. Aching in region of eye, with photophobia and lachrymation, ameliorated in a dark room and toward noon. Evenings at six o'clock, aching pain in region of eyes and pinching in the eyes, ameliorated by lachrymation. In open air itching in eyes, must frequently wink and wipe them, with lachrymation. Photophobia.

Clinical. Euphrasia is one of our most important remedies in diseases of the eye, especially superficial; its sphere of action is well defined, but its indiscriminate use (as employed by many practitioners) in all cases of ophthalmia is not to be imitated.

In blepharitis it has proved very valuable, as the result of many cases show; the lids are red, swollen and covered with a thick yellow acrid discharge, often mixed with the profuse, acrid, burning lachrymation, which makes the lids and cheek sore and excoriated, and is frequently accompanied by fluent coryza; firm agglutination of the lids in the morning.

The cases of catarrhal and strumous inflammation of the cornea and conjunctiva, which speedily respond to this drug, are to be counted by scores, for it is in these cases that Euphrasia is especially adapted. Useful in both the chronic and acute form of inflammation, but especially in the latter:—Catarrhal inflammation from exposure to the cold; catarrhal inflammation of the eyes and nose in the first stage of measles; papillary trachoma, with or without pannus; pustules on the cornea and conjunctiva; superficial ulceration of the cornea (sometimes accompanied with pannus), though is rarely indicated in the deep form, except, perhaps, as a palliative in the first stage. In all the above cases we usually find much photophobia, though it may be nearly absent; the lachrymation is profuse, acrid, and burning, as well as the thick, yellow, muco-purulent discharge, which is usually present and excoriates the lids, making them red, inflamed and sore, as well as giving the cheek an appearance as if varnished. The conjunctiva may be quite red, even to chemosis. The pains are not marked, though usually of a smarting, sticking, or burning character, from the nature of the discharges. Fluent coryza often accompanies the above symptoms.

Blurring of the eyes relieved by winking, so often found in superficial inflammations of the eye, due to the secretions getting upon the cornea, thus interfering with vision and then carried away by the movement of the lids in winking, is a simple symptom, which is almost invariably relieved by Euphrasia.

Purulent ophthalmia has been benefited, particularly that form found in new-born children (ophthalmia neonatorum); the symptoms given above indicate its choice and are seen to call for its use more often in the later stages, than at the commencement of the disease.

Opacities of the cornea, resulting from repeated attacks of inflammation, are reported cured by several observers.

Several cases of rheumatic iritis are on record, as speedily relieved by this drug, in which there was great ciliary injection, photophobia, dimness of the aqueous, discoloration of the iris, posterior synechiæ and constant aching, with occasional darting pain in the eye, always worse at night.

The following case illustrates its usefulness in paralysis of the muscles:—A man, æt. 52, appeared for treatment, with total paralysis of the oculo-motor nerve, even to those filaments which supply the iris and ciliary muscle; came on rapidly after exposure in the cold and wet. Electricity was applied every day or two for about five weeks, and either Rhus or Caust. given internally at the same time, with no benefit. At the end of this time, on account of some slight catarrhal symptoms, Euphras.^{30} was given and the electricity continued. After taking two doses of Euphras., the upper lid began to rise, the pupil to contract and the eye to move inward; and within four weeks a complete cure was effected.

Euphrasia is very similar to Mercurius in the character of

its discharges, only that in Merc. they are thin and excoriating, while under Euphras. they are thick and excoriating. Arsen. also has acrid secretions, but they are usually thin, not as profuse as the above remedies and accompanied by much burning pain, photophobia, etc. Rhus, like Euphras., has profuse lachrymation, but it is not as excoriating. In paralysis of the muscles, caused from exposure to cold or wet, Euphras. may be compared to Caust. and Rhus, the remedies upon which we chiefly rely in these affections, but is especially called for when a catarrhal condition of the eye is, at the same time, present.

FERRUM.

Clinical. Ferrum jodatus is the form of iron, which has been more commonly employed in diseases of the eye.

A case of scrofulous inflammation of the eyes:—Eyes shut on account of pain and photophobia; lids swollen, copious discharge of pus on forcibly opening; conjunctiva bluish-red and swollen; skin pale; nose thick; eczema of face; sub-maxillary and cervical glands swollen and hard; periostitis of one finger and two toes; body emaciated; abdomen large and no appetite; is reported cured, after Bell. had failed, by Fischer in A. H. Z.

Has been used by Dr. Liebold with great benefit in exophthalmic goitre. One case occurred in a woman after suppression of the menses, characterized by protrusion of the eyes, enlargement of the thyroid gland, palpitation of the heart and excessive nervousness. Ferr. jod. was given when the menses soon reappeared, the nervousness diminished and all the symptoms improved. Another similar case occurring in a colored woman, was relieved by the acetate of iron.

FLUORIC ACID.

Sensation as if strong cold wind were blowing in the eyes, must tie them up and keep them warm.

Clinical. A case of lachrymal fistula of the left side, of one year's duration; a clear yellow scab on the cheek near the inner angle, which is only a little red and painful to pressure; every three or four days it begins to itch and grow moist, then heads again; sometimes painful before it opens. Fluoric acid^{30}, cured.—HERING.

GELSEMIUM.

Objective. Paralysis of the lids. Heaviness, impossible to raise the lids. Constant inclination to squint.

Subjective. Heat in eyes and forehead. Bruised pain above and behind the eyes. Soreness as from a foreign body, no pain, with photophobia and lachrymation.

Aggravation of eye symptoms from the use of wine.

Vision. Diplopia, can correct it by his will. Diplopia on looking sideways. Diplopia in pregnancy. Dim vision during pregnancy. Swimming black specks before eyes, vision dim, can neither read nor write, words run together, cannot recognize one across the room, with heat in eyes extending to forehead. As if a snake were before vision with pain over the eyes. Blindness with dilated pupils. Photophobia.

Clinical. Gelsemium is rarely found of benefit in superficial affections of the eye, but is especially adapted to diseases of the fundus and paralysis of the nerves.

Ptosis, coming on after an attack of ophthalmia, (which yielded to Acon. and Euphras.) was cured in forty-eight hours by Gels.^{2}.—GALLINGER.

Paralysis of the oculo-motor and of the abducens have been benefited and the resulting diplopia relieved. Diplopia with spasm of various muscles throughout the body, without thirst, was quickly cured.

In inflammatory affections of the retina and choroid, it is particularly useful.

Retinitis albuminurica, in which the dimness of vision came on suddenly during pregnancy, worse after delivery, with no pain, only an itching of the eyes; white patches and extravasations of blood are to be seen in the retina, while the outer part of the optic nerve appears whiter than usual. Recovery took place under Gels.

Chorio-retinitis, in which there seemed to be a bluish snake before the vision, was cured.

In serous choroiditis it is an excellent remedy, especially if the haziness of the vitreous is very fine, tension increased, pupils dilated, much soreness of the eyeball to touch, aching pain over and in the eyes, and if the vision varies greatly in a short time, being one day very dim and the next quite bright. A case, occurring in a woman, æt. 50, dark complexion and bilious temperament, with all the above symptoms and decided hyperæmia of the optic nerve and retina, was treated some six weeks with several remedies, (chiefly Bry.) with varying success. At last in addition to these symptoms, small transparent points made their appearance on the right cornea, looking like the swollen ends of nerve filaments, and were excessively sensitive to touch or any movement of the lid; they would come and go suddenly, often in the same day; after two days they became permanent and were very painful. Gels.^{30} was given, when they gradually disappeared, the vitreous cleared and the vision was completely restored within two weeks.

Amaurosis appearing in a woman, æt. 45, after an attack of "putrid sore throat:"—Pupils of both eyes dilated and iris sluggish; vision nearly lost; the right palate was slightly paralyzed and the uvula deviated to the left; is on record as cured.—J. L. Newton.

In paralysis of the nerves, compare Gels. with Caust., Con. and Rhus; and in serous choroiditis, compare with Bryonia.

The condition which indicates Gels., is usually one of stolid indifference to external irritants, in which respect it stands in marked contrast to Conium, whose paralytic symptoms are characterized by great reflex, irritability, (photophobia, etc).

In detachment of the retina Gels. is very commonly indicated and great benefit has been seen from its use.

GRAPHITES.

Objective. Redness and painful inflammation of lower lid and internal canthus. Inflammation of external canthus. Margins of lids much inflamed. Dry hardened mucus in the lashes. Redness of the white of the eye, with lachrymation and photophobia.

Subjective. Itching in internal canthus. Sense of dryness in the lids and pressure. Biting pain in the eyes as from something acrid. Heat in the eyes and some matter in the canthi. Heat in the eyes with indistinct vision. Biting in the eyes with heat.

Photophobia, especially by daylight.

Clinical. We have few remedies in the materia medica so commonly indicated in inflammatory conditions of the lids, conjunctiva and cornea, as Graphites, especially if occurring in scrofulous subjects with eczematous eruptions, which are moist, fissured, bleed easily and are situated chiefly on the head and behind the ears.

It is chiefly indicated in the chronic form of blepharitis or in eczema of the lids, though sometimes called for in acute attacks, particularly if complicated with such affections of the cornea as ulcers and pustules. In chronic ciliary blepharitis in which Graphites is useful, the edges of the lids will usually be found slightly swollen and of a pale red color; the inflammation may be confined to the canthi (blepharitis angularis), *especially to the outer, which have a great tendency to crack and bleed easily* upon any attempt to open them; the margins may be ulcerated; *dry scurfs are usually present on the ciliæ;* there is burning and dryness in the lids, biting and itching, causing a constant desire to rub them.

In eczema of the lids, the eruption will be found moist and fissured, while the margins of the lids are covered with scales or crusts.

Tarsal tumors, especially cystic, have been removed by this remedy.

In catarrhal ophthalmia, Graphites has been employed with

benefit, but in scrofulous ophthalmia, characterized by ulcers and pustules, it is second to no other drug in importance. It has cured deep ulcers of the cornea even with hypopion, but it is more particularly adapted to superficial ulcerations, especially if resulting from pustules, often with considerable vascularity of the cornea. The pustules which have been removed under the influence of Graphites, have been of various kinds and accompanied by varying symptoms; they may be either on the cornea or conjunctiva, but especially on the former; the attacks may be acute or chronic, but it is particularly called for in the chronic recurrent form.

The following case illustrates very markedly the action of this remedy:—A boy had been troubled for a long time with chronic pustular inflammation of the cornea, no sooner would he recover from one attack before another would appear; there was great photophobia so that he could not open his eyes to see his way, profuse lachrymation, burning and aching in the eyes, sneezing upon opening them, *external canthi cracked and easily bleeding*, both corneæ pannoused, thin acrid discharge from the eyes, and *nose sore and surrounded by thick moist scabs.* Under the use of Graph. a rapid and permanent cure was effected.

The *photophobia is usually intense* and the lachrymation profuse, though in some cases nearly or entirely absent; is generally worse by daylight than gaslight, and in the morning, so that often the child cannot open the eyes before 9 or 10 A.M. The redness of the eye is generally marked and the discharges of a muco-purulent character, constant, thin and excoriating. The pains are not important and vary; may be of a sticking, burning, aching or itching character. The lids are red, sore and agglutinated in the morning, or else covered with *dry scurfs*, and the *external canthi are cracked and bleed easily* upon opening the eye (this is the most characteristic symptom under the drug).

We very often notice a thin acrid discharge from the nose accompanying the ophthalmias of Graph.

Graphites is somewhat similar to Hepar and Sulphur in

scrofulous inflammation of the eyes. But under Graphites the discharges from the eyes and nose are more thin and excoriating, and there is a greater tendency towards cracking of the external canthi. The latter symptom is also sometimes observed under Hepar, but is not as marked, while the discharge is not as excoriating, lids more swollen, eye more red and ulceration deeper. The Sulphur patient is more restless and feverish at night, and complains of occasional sharp sticking pains in the eye, while the face and body may be covered with eruptions, which, however, differ in character from that of Graph.

HAMAMELIS VIRGINICA.

Clinical. A spontaneous eversion of the upper lid during the course of a severe conjunctivitis, was relieved by the application of dilute "Pond's Extract."—W. S. Searle.

Dr. Holcombe reported a case several years ago of traumatic conjunctivitis from the burn of a flame, which caused excruciating pain, great photophobia, constant acrid lachrymation and great vascularity of the conjunctiva. Ham. virg., 30 drops to an ounce of water, applied externally, gave immediate relief and cured the case. Another case is also reported of conjunctivitis traumatica from a piece of splinter under the upper lid, in which Ham. produced prompt relief.

This remedy has been employed with excellent success in many cases of inflammation of the conjunctiva and cornea, even in ulceration of the latter, if caused from a blow or burn.

Marked results have been obtained from its use in hastening the absorption of hemorrhages in the anterior chamber.

A case of traumatic iritis, with great pain at night and hemorrhage into the interior of the eye, was speedily relieved.

HEPAR SULPHUR.

Objective. Redness, inflammation and swelling of upper lid, with pressive pain. Papular eruption on upper lids and under eyes. Inflammation and swelling of eyelids, with redness of whites. Lachrymation.

Subjective. Boring pain in roof of orbits. Smarting pain in external canthus, with accumulation of hard mucus. Pressive pain in eyeballs and as if beaten on touch. Pressure in eyes worse on moving, with redness. Pressure in eyes with lachrymation.

Photophobia.

Clinical. Hepar is useful in certain forms of blepharitis in which the lids are inflamed, sore and corroded, as if eaten, or when small red swellings are found along the margins of the lids, which are painful in the evening and on touch, with itching pimples on the face; also called for if the meibomian glands are affected.

It is, however, in acute phlegmonous inflammation of the lids, which tend towards suppuration, that this remedy is particularly valuable; the lids are inflamed as if erysipelas had invaded them, with *throbbing*, aching, stinging pain, and are very *sensitive to touch;* the pains are aggravated by cold and *relieved by warmth.* In fact, for abscesses of the lids, it is the most commonly indicated remedy.

Eczema of the lids, in which thick honey comb scabs are found both on and around the lids, with nocturnal agglutination, etc., is especially amenable to Hepar.

Palpebral tumors have disappeared under its use.

For dacryocystitis and orbital cellulitis, after pus has formed, Hepar should be always borne in mind, as it is very useful indeed, according to the potency administered, either producing absorption or accelerating the discharge.

In catarrhal ophthalmia is often useful, but in the severer forms of strumous ophthalmia, in which the pustules and ulcers are situated on the cornea and marked by the intensity of the symptoms, there is probably no remedy more frequently indicated than Hepar.

Pustules on the conjunctiva uncomplicated with corneal disease, rarely call for this drug.

It is chiefly indicated in ulcers and abscesses of the cornea, especially in the deep sloughing form of ulcer if complicated with hypopion. It has proved curative in some torpid ulcers when general symptoms have pointed to its use, but there is usually *intense photophobia*, *profuse lachrymation*, *great redness of the cornea and conjunctiva* even to chemosis, and *much pain* of a *throbbing*, aching, shooting character, which is *relieved by warmth*, so that one constantly wishes to keep the eye covered, is worse on any draught of air (Sil.) and at night or in the evening; the lids are often swollen, spasmodically closed and very *sensitive to touch*, or may be red, swollen and *bleed easily upon opening*.

Has been employed very successfully in cases of trachoma with pannus, in which the pannus has taken on an acute form and tends toward ulceration; especially indicated in mercurialized subjects.

"Hepar is the main remedy for keratitis punctata."—Payr.

In keratitis parenchymatosa it serves to promote resorption after the disease has been checked by Merc., Aurum, Calc. or other remedies.

Benefit has been derived from its use in opacities of the cornea.

Many cases of kerato-iritis have been cured, as the following case will illustrate:—A man was attacked with severe inflammation in the cornea and iris of the left eye; cornea ulcerated superficially, much ciliary injection, pupil contracted, iris sluggish, great photophobia and lachrymation, much pain extending from the eye into the corresponding side of the head, worse at night, especially about two or three A.M.; seat of pain in the head, as well as the eye, quite sore to touch; lids considerably swollen and slight discharge. Hepar cured in a short time.

Iritis, particularly if accompanied with hypopion, is often controlled by this drug.

For the absorption of pus in the anterior chamber (hypopion), there is no better remedy than Hepar.

From its usefulness in hypopion and suppurative inflammations in general, it has been administered, with benefit in inflammations of a part or whole of the uveal tract, if, of a suppurative tendency.

Bojanus reports, in A. H. Z., a case of complete amaurosis, pupils dilated and insensible to light, resulting from enormous doses of mercury, in which the sight was restored under the use of Hepar.

Ulceration of external parts of the eye, which bleed easily and are very sensitive to touch, most positively indicate Hepar. These cases usually suffer from excessive photophobia, which is also very marked under Merc. protiod., whilst Kali bichrom., though indicated in extensive destruction of tissue and great sensitiveness of the eye to touch, lacks entirely the photophobia so marked under Hepar.

HYOSCYAMUS.

Twitchings in the eye. Dim vision, as if a veil before the eyes. Objects appear red and too large. Farsightedness, with very clear vision and dilated pupils.

Clinical. Hyoscyamus has relieved the excessive photophobia, occurring in scrofulous ophthalmia.—GARAY.

Hoppe reports a case of iritis, supervening upon ulceration of the cornea in a scrofulous child, nine months old; conjunctiva injected; cornea dim, bluish and ulcerated in one spot, after a pustule; iris discolored, much pain at night. Hyosc.[3] cured.

Convergent squint of the right eye, occurring in a girl, twelve years of age, due to spasmodic action of the internal rectus muscle; eye turned in so much that only one-half of the pupil could be seen, was cured by Hyos.[3].—GALLAVARDIN. Another case of convergent squint, due to paresis of the abducens, is reported cured by the same author, with Hyos. 30th and 200th. There was in this case diplopia, everything appeared as if in a cloud and too large, with drawing pains in the right eyeball, brow and forehead; it was thought to have a rheumatic origin.

Several cases of hemeralopia have been cured by this remedy: —One case occurred in a young man after intermittent fever and was of high degree; pupils dilated, distant objects seen better than near.—Löscher. Another case found in a myopic eye, with shooting pains from the eyes into the nose and head; headache ameliorated on closing the eyes, was relieved by Hyosc.

IGNATIA.

In the evening the inner surface of the upper lid pains as if it were too dry. In external canthus of left eye, sensation as if dust were in it. Evenings on reading, it seems dim before the eye as from tears which he should wipe away, but there are none. Lachrymation and photophobia.

Clinical. Morbid nictitation, with spasmodic action of various muscles of the face, has been relieved.

Ignatia has been employed with benefit in traumatic ophthalmia, with violent pains and sensation as if sand were rolling around beneath the lids; also in catarrhal ophthalmia, with a sensation of sand in the eye and great dryness, lachrymation only in the sunlight.

A case of ciliary neuralgia, in a woman, was cured very promptly by this remedy; the pains were very severe, extending from the eye to the top of the head, producing nausea, and often alternated with swelling in the throat (globus hystericus); the pains would begin very slightly, increase gradually until they became very severe, and would only cease when she became exhausted.

Asthenopia and amblyopia found in females, due to onanism, have been helped by Ignatia.

IPECACUANHA.

Constrictive pain over the orbit and in the left temple. Pain pressing out and almost boring in a small spot, now over the orbit, now in temples, ameliorated by external pressure and closing the eyes.

Clinical. Ciliary neuralgia is said to have been relieved.

The following symptoms observed in a patient, are reported in the Brit. Journ. of Hom., as relieved by Ipecac.[12]:—A woman, æt. 47, was suffering from severe shooting pains through the eyeballs, profuse lachrymation on looking steadily, blue and red halo around flame, pupil normal and mobile, with no external inflammation or lesion, except slight palpebral conjunctivitis.

KALI ACETICUM.

Clinical. Amaurosis coming on suddenly in both eyes, in a patient suffering from acute nephritis. Vision was restored by this form of potash.—WINDELBAND.

KALI BICHROMICUM.

Clinical. The following case of trachoma with pannus, was as near cured as it possibly could be:—A man, æt. 27, had granular lids, complete pannus of right eye so could barely count fingers, and partial pannus of the left eye; there was considerable discharge and everything appeared slightly red to him; eyes seemed to feel better when lying on the face. Under Kali bichrom. the pannus entirely cleared, leaving a slight opacity behind, but could read No. 3 Snellen's test type easily with the right eye.

It is of especial importance, however, in chronic indolent forms of inflammation of the eye, particularly of ulcers and pustules on the cornea, in which no active inflammatory process is present, and therefore characterized by *no photophobia and no redness*, or very little, not as much as might be expected from the nature of the disease; the pains and lachrymation are also usually absent. The eye is often quite sensitive to touch and its secretions are of a *stringy character*.

Opacities of the cornea have frequently been benefited and even cleared up entirely under the use of Kali bichrom. Sometimes used internally alone, and again both externally and internally at the same time.

Rheumatic sclero-iritis in a syphilitic subject, with excessive pain and photophobia, is reported cured by Drysdale.

KALI CARBONICUM.

Redness and vascularity of the white of the eye. Inflammation of lids of right eye, with pain in the eyes and impossibility to read by light. Swelling between the brow and lid, like a sack. Lachrymation.

Soreness of external canthus with burning pain. Stitches and smarting in eyes and lids. Painful sensitiveness of eyes to daylight.

Clinical. Œdema of the lids, especially if accompanied by sticking pains and heart indications, often subsides under the use of Kali carb.

Occasionally called for in blepharitis, as the following will illustrate:—A sewing woman, æt. 60, has frequently suffered from arthritic pains, and now the eyelids are swollen, edges and canthi red, caruncula red and swollen, with lachrymation and pain in bright light; there is also pressing pain from forehead and temples into the eye, with heat in the face and head, loss of appetite, pressure in the stomach after eating, nausea and sensation of emptiness in the stomach, retching and vomiting of mucus, pressure and anxious feeling in the chest, chilliness, cold feet, evening fever with thirst, weariness and heaviness in the limbs, face pale, dirty gray, restless sleep and a great deal of yawning through the day. Kali carb.[3], three doses cured in a few days.—J. SCHELLING.

In small round ulcers of the cornea with no photophobia, the carbonate of potash has been used with benefit.

Pannus always worse after a seminal emission, has been removed by this drug.

The following case of asthenopia was relieved by Kali carb.[6]:—A young lady, eighteen years of age, was troubled with sticking and drawing together of the lids upon looking steadily at any object; if she persisted in using them, a burning pressing pain in the eyes would be experienced; on the slightest exertion the borders of the lids would become red and swollen, palpebral fissure narrowed and palpebral conjunctiva hyperæmic; constant photophobia was present, so was compelled to keep the eyes closed most of the time, always worse after using them; no abnormal appearances could be detected. Slight rheumatism. Health good.—KAFKA.

KALI IODATUM.

Clinical. The iodide of potash has produced pustules on the cornea and conjunctiva, when given in massive and long continued doses, and has cured cases in which no photophobia, pain or redness were present. In this respect does not differ from the bichromate.

Sometimes useful in stricture of the lachrymal duct.

Is often indicated in iritis (syphilitic) especially after mercurialization. In paralysis of the muscles dependent upon syphilitic periostitis, the iodide of potash is the remedy most frequently called for, no matter which muscle is affected.

Is one of our most important drugs for irido-choroiditis, acute or chronic, and choroiditis disseminata, especially if of syphilitic origin. The special indications are not known, though its effects are often marvelous, as the following case of disseminate choroiditis, occurring in a young lady, not syphilitic and accompanied by occasional headaches, will illustrate:—The fundus of the right eye showed extensive white patches (atrophy of the choroid) and deposits of pigment over its whole extent, optic nerve hyperæmic, slight haziness of the vitreous. Commencing atrophic spots in the choroid of the left eye and hyperæmia of the nerve, could be detected by the ophthalmoscope. R. v. $\frac{20}{200}$ L. v. $\frac{20}{20}$. She was directed not to use the eyes more than necessary, and Bell. was given for three or four weeks with no marked improvement, with this exception, that the headaches were not quite as frequent. Kali iod.[1] was now prescribed, when the eyes rapidly began to grow stronger, the hyperæmia of the fundus disappeared and the headaches ceased entirely. Six months after using Kali iod., R. v. $\frac{20}{30}$ L. v. $\frac{20}{20}$, though the atrophic spots in the choroid, of course, underwent no change.

KALI MURIATICUM.

Clinical. The following case, described by Dr. Woodyatt, shows that it must be an important remedy in intra-ocular troubles:—Chorio-retinitis. Mr. D., æt. 36. Noticed two years ago such dimness of the right eye, that he could not read a newspaper. Had observed no previous trouble. After a month's treatment he could read again, but suffering a relapse, the same treatment for a year proved ineffectual and the case was deemed hopeless. No history of syphilis. Examination showed cornea, iris and pupil normal. No external redness. By ophthalmoscope: Vitreous rather hazy, with some black shreds suspended in it, having very limited motion on rotating the eye. This would indicate that the vitreous was not fluid. Optic nerve and blood-vessels normal. Inside the disk, a large, irregular, atrophic spot, involving the choroid and retina, surrounded by several small ones; edges irregular and pigmented; the sclerotic seen white through their centres; choroid adjacent, congested and thickened; some vessels lost in the infiltrated part to appear on the other side; a dull pain, occasionally, in the eye and over the brow, with an ill-defined feeling of contraction around the eye. Vision $\frac{20}{200}$. Snellen 11 slowly deciphered. Prescribed Kali mur. 6th dec., four times daily. At the end of a month vision rose to $\frac{20}{50}$ and snellen 3 was read at five inches. A year afterwards the man could read snellen $2\frac{1}{2}$, distant vision $\frac{20}{70}$, but under Kali mur., for a week, it was again $\frac{20}{50}$. The patient's business engagements prevented longer treatment.

KALMIA LATIFOLIA.

Sensation of stiffness in the muscles around the eyes and of the eyelids. Glimmering before the eyes, exactly in the point of vision. Everything becomes black before the eyes on looking down, with nausea and eructations of wind, worse in the morning from eight to nine o'clock.

Clinical. From its action upon the muscles we are led to give it in asthenopia, and with good results, especially if there is present a *stiff drawing sensation in the muscles* upon moving the eyes.

Sclero-choroiditis ant., in which the sclera was inflamed, vitreous perfectly filled with exudations and glimmering of light before the eye, especially on reading with the other, was cured by this drug.

Kalmia was prescribed in a case of retinitis albuminurica, occurring during pregnancy, on account of the characteristic pains in the back; it was continued for a long time, during which the white patches gradually became absorbed and recovery took place.

KREOSOTUM.

Lachrymation; discharge of hot, acrid, smarting tears, like salt water, worse in a bright light, on rubbing the eyes and early in the morning. Itching, biting and smarting in the eyes.

Clinical. Has been of service in acute aggravations of chronic keratitis, in which there is excessive, hot, smarting lachrymation; also in blennorrhœa of the conjunctiva, with moderately profuse discharge and much smarting in the eyes.

LACHESIS.

Inflammations of the eyes and lids, with pain in them. A variety of stitching, burning and pressing pains in the eyes.

Sharp, shooting pains from eyes (left eye) to temples, top of head and occiput.

Dimness of vision on first waking. Mistiness and flickering before the eyes.

Clinical. Scrofulous keratitis with eruption on the face, considerable photophobia and pains in the eye and head, worse in the morning and *after sleeping*, is frequently very quickly relieved by Lachesis.

Orbital cellulitis, following an operation for strabismus; eye protruded; conjunctiva chemosed; purulent discharge; retina hazy and congested; point of tenotomy sloughing and a black spot in the center; worse at night; was effectually and rapidly cured by this remedy.

The snake poisons, as suggested by Dr. Liebold, but particularly Lachesis, are the best and most commonly indicated remedies we possess for retinitis apoplectica. We have used it in several cases of hemorrhage into the retina with brilliant results, whether of spontaneous origin or dependent upon various diseased conditions of the fundus.

It seems not only to hasten very materially the absorption of any hemorrhage into the retina, but also to control the inflammatory symptoms and diminish the tendency to retinal extravasations.

LACTIC ACID.

Clinical. Hyperæsthesia of the retina, with steady aching pain in and behind the eyeball, was quickly relieved by a few doses of Lactic acid.

LEDUM PALUSTRE.

Clinical. Ecchymoses of the conjunctiva, either of traumatic or spontaneous origin, are often quickly absorbed by the use of this remedy, and in many cases more promptly than when our usual remedies, Arnica or Hamamelis, are employed. (Should be used in the same manner as Arnica.)

The following interesting case of rheumatic ophthalmia is reported cured with Ledum, by Franz Alb, in A. H. Z.:—A man, æt. 49; the left eye became first affected, after which it extended to the right; there was excessive photophobia, with severe pain upon attempting to open the lids, and pressing pain in the head and eyes, as if it at first were pressed assunder, then out of the orbit, with great lachrymation and nocturnal aggravation; severe burning on the border of the lids and sticking in the eyes, as from sand; tearing, drawing pains in the neck to the insertion of the deltoid muscle; heat and chills were also present.

LITHIUM CARBONICUM.

On reading, pain as if the eyes were dry and ailing. Hemiopia, right half invisible, with pain over eye and a tension as if bound in temples.

Clinical. Asthenopia, with black motes before the eyes and sensitiveness of the eyes after using them by candle-light, has been relieved.

In hemiopia, in which only the left half of the field of vision is present, Lithium seems especially indicated. Dr. Dunham reports such a case, in which only the left half of an object was visible with the right eye, and nothing at all with the left. Lith. carb.^{30} made a brilliant cure.

(Two or three cases of hemiopia, in which the left half of objects was visible, have been treated by Lithium without success.—Eds.)

LYCOPODIUM.

Objective. Inflammation of eyes, with itching in canthi; redness and swelling of lids; troublesome pain if they were dry, and nightly agglutination. Pustules and styes on lids, especially towards the inner canthus. Much mucus in the eyes, with smarting pain. Lachrymation severe afternoons.

Vision. On writing, letters become indistinct. Floating black spots before the eyes. Like a veil and flickering before the eyes after the afternoon nap. Hemiopia, he sees only the left half of objects, right half is unseen or only dim, with one eye as with both; (all this is worse in right eye).

Clinical. But few external diseases have been cured by this drug; its chief remedial power has been exhibited in disorders of nutrition and function of the deep-seated structures of the eye.

Ciliary blepharitis and hordeola, occasionally call for the use of this drug when the general symptoms indicate.

Polypus at the external canthus, as large as a sweet pea, was cured in fourteen days by Lyco.[200].—GROSS. (Another case of polypus in the inner canthus of the right eye, was not in the slightest degree affected by Lyco.—EDS.)

Dimness of the lens (?) especially in the right eye, occurring after an attack of typhus and suppression of the menses. Under Lyco.[4], the menses appeared in a few days, and soon afterward the sight was restored.—DIEZ.

The following symptoms occurring in a man, sixty years of age, are reported by Hilberger:—During writing the vision would suddenly disappear, as if a dark cloud passed before the sight, so that only large objects could be seen; vision better in the forenoon and in the open air; the sclera was injected, pupil contracted and fundus hazy. Headache and congestion of the liver were present. Cured by Lyco.[6].

Opacities in the vitreous have occasionally been known to disappear during the administration of Lyco.

In hemeralopia, its great value as an eye remedy becomes apparent, for no other drug in our materia medica has cured such a large number of cases as Lyco. There seems to be no marked indication for its use, with the exception of the night blindness coming on in the early eve, though in some instances it was found that the patient could see better at a distance than near at hand, yet in other cases this indication was wanting, so it cannot be considered important. If black spots floating before the eyes accompany the night blindness, this drug is particularly called for.

Hemiopia, in which the right half of the field of vision is obscured, has been restored.

Progress of cataract arrested by Lyco., prescribed for chronic dyspeptic symptoms.

LYCOPUS VIRGINICUS.

Clinical. This remedy will doubtless prove of great importance in the treatment of exophthalmic goitre (morbus Basedowii) though on account of its comparatively recent addition to our materia medica, it has not been very extensively employed, yet cases have been relieved and some are said to have been cured.

MAGNESIA CARBONICA.

Clinical. Rückert advises its use from experience in scrofulous ophthalmia, with opacities on the cornea.

Cases of cataract in which the diagnosis seems to have been very clear, are reported cured by several authors.

MANGANUM.

Clinical. Asthenopia, with aching pains in the eyes on looking at near objects, so must close them; still worse on looking at a near light, was speedily relieved.

MERCURIUS CYANURET.

Clinical. The Cyanuret of Mercury has been employed with benefit in kerato-iritis syphilitica, in which there has been much inflammation and severe nocturnal pains.—NUNEZ. But there seems to be no characteristic symptoms to distinguish it from the other forms of Mercury in more common use.

MERCURIUS DULCIS.

Clinical. Calomel has been employed for many years by the old school in scrofulous ophthalmia, and even to this day it is considered by them, one of their most important remedies, though not a specific, as was formerly supposed. Dusting the fine powder in the eye, is the manner in which it is used by them.

We, also, as homœopaths, find it adapted to certain forms of strumous ophthalmia, though given in a different manner, in different doses and upon different principles. We use it only internally and for the general cachexia, as the following case will illustrate:—A little girl, æt. 6, light complexion, pale skin, muscles soft and flabby, glands enlarged and general strumous diathesis. Upon examination, a very deep ulcer was found on the left cornea, which had so nearly perforated that the membrane of descemet had begun to bulge; small ulcers and pustules were present on the border of the cornea. In the right eye, pustules and maculæ were also seen on the cornea. There was considerable redness and great photophobia. Various remedies, chiefly the anti-psorics, had been given with no benefit. Merc. dulc.^{2}, three doses daily, was now administered, when improvement soon began and went rapidly on to recovery, leaving only a macula behind.

Benefit has also been derived from the use of Merc. dulc. in deeper forms of inflammation of the eye, as in irido-choroiditis, etc., especially if dependent upon a scrofulous diathesis, and the general cachexia of the patient suggests the remedy.

MERCURIUS NITRAS.

Clinical. This preparation of Mercury has been used successfully, both externally and internally, in various forms of blepharitis marked by no particular indications.

But it is especially adapted to scrofulous ophthalmia, in which ulcers and pustules are present, particularly the latter, and has been used, especially by Dr. Liebold, with remarkable success in a large number of cases without regard to symptoms. Severe cases, as well as mild, chronic cases, as well as acute and superficial, as well as deep (even with hypopion), have yielded to its influence; also in some cases there has been much photophobia, in others none at all; in some severe pain, while in others it has been absent, and thus we might go through a variety of other symptoms, differing as much as the above, in which this drug has been curative. It is employed both externally and internally at the same time and in the lower potencies, say about the first potency, ten grains to two drams of water (or even stronger) as an external application, to be used in the eye, two, three or more times a day, and the second or third potency to be taken internally. Atropine is sometimes used with it, especially if there is much photophobia present.

MERCURIUS PRÆCIPITATUS RUBER.

Clinical. The red precipitate of Mercury so often used by the old school, has been too little employed by us, as we have no symptomatology, but are guided in its selection simply by clinical indications.

In scrofulous ophthalmia it has proved very beneficial; there is commonly bright red swelling of the conjunctiva, often so great as to evert the lids; granulations are frequently present; the cornea is superficially ulcerated and covered with red vessels; the discharges from the eye are copious and purulent, forming crusts upon the lids, which are firmly agglutinated in the morning; the photophobia is usually great.

Benefit has been derived from its use in ophthalmia neonatorum.

In trachoma, with pannus, it is a valuable remedy, rarely, however, of much use in acute cases, but seems especially adapted to old chronic cases, in which the cornea is covered with pannus of high degree, with considerable redness, discharge and photophobia; granulations may be present, or may have been already removed by caustics.

MERCURIUS PROTOIODATUS.

Clinical. In some cases of blepharitis of syphilitic origin good results have been obtained from Merc. prot., if the concomitant symptoms point to its use.

Trachoma with and without pannus has been followed by marked improvement.

Pustular inflammation of the cornea and conjunctiva has been removed, but its principal sphere of action is in ulceration of the cornea; chiefly in that form of ulceration that commences at the margin of the cornea and *extends, involving only the superficial layers, either over the whole cornea or a portion of it, particularly the upper part*, which appears as if chipped out with the finger nail, the so-called serpiginous form; also in cases of *ulceration occurring in the course of pannus and granular conjunctivitis*, it is excelled by no other remedy in frequency of indication.

In all these cases there is usually present excessive photophobia and redness, though sometimes these may be nearly absent. The pains are generally of a throbbing, aching character and worse at night; the pain often extends up into the head, which is sore to touch. In nearly every case we have the *thick yellow coating at the base of the tongue* and swelling of the glands in various parts of the body, which are so prominent under this drug.

Is often indicated in pannus, especially in acute aggravations.

Cases of paralysis of the oculo-motor nerve of syphilitic origin have been restored to power by this preparation of mercury.

In intra-ocular troubles, Dr. Woodyatt has observed very favorable results from the use of the iodide of mercury, as in opacities of the vitreous and in irido-choroiditis, as the following will illustrate:—"Miss L., aged 26. Eight years ago noticed a drooping and heaviness of eyelids. After two years found sight of left eye imperfect, and when this dimness appeared, the drooping of both eyelids ceased. No redness, pain, nor photophobia; but black spots and flashes of light were sometimes seen. A year later, the right eye was affected and rapidly grew worse than the left. Two years ago the sight failed entirely. Examination of right eye: no external redness; anterior chamber shallow; iris discolored, and crowded forward by a swollen opaque lens, to the capsule of which it was attached all around the margin of a contracted pupil. Not even quantitative sight existed. Left eye: anterior chamber shallow; iris dimmed and discolored; pupil moderately dilated and mobile. Ophthalmoscope revealed pigment spots on the lens capsule; vitreous hazy throughout; lying in it, near the retina, three greenish blue spots, a little larger than the optic nerve; probably hemorrhagic effusions undergoing degeneration. Vision $\frac{20}{60}$. Snellen $1\frac{1}{2}$ read slowly at three inches; irregular dilatation of pupil under Atropine. Patient in fair health and only complains of black spots in the visual axis, inability to bear strong light and to use her eyes continuously. Prescribed Mercurius iod., 3d dec., four times a day; to use protective glasses and to abstain from 'near work.' Twenty days later vision $\frac{20}{30}$. Snellen $1\frac{1}{2}$ read at eight inches. During the menses, two days after this record, there was hemorrhage into the vitreous. For one day, sight was only quantitative, but it rapidly cleared. For ten days, vision $\frac{20}{20}$ emmetropic. Résumé: Duration of treatment, 60 days; left eye; vision from $\frac{20}{60}$ to $\frac{20}{20}$."

MERCURIUS SOLUBIS.

Objective. Great swelling, redness and constriction of the lids; they are sensitive to touch. The upper lid is thick and red, like a stye. Lids agglutinated mornings. Congestion in white of eye. Inflammatory swelling in region of lachrymal bone.

The eyes close forcibly, whether sitting, standing or walking.

Subjective. Burning and heat in the eye, with lachrymation. Aching and itching in the eye. Aching in the eye on motion or touch. Burning sensation in the right brow.

Vision. Black muscæ volitantes constantly flit before sight. Cloud before one or both eyes. Fiery sparks before the eyes. Letters seem to move in the evening on reading. Firelight at evening blinds exceedingly. Cannot endure firelight or daylight.

Clinical. Mercury, this form in particular, has been one of our chief remedies in ophthalmic practice for many years and even now it may be considered one of our polychrests. Its range of action is, however, circumscribed, but well marked.

In blepharitis there is no better remedy, if the lids are *red, thick and swollen* (particularly the upper), and sensitive to heat, cold or touch; the lachrymation is *profuse, burning and acrid*, making the lids sore, red and painful, especially worse in the open air, or by the constant application of cold water; the symptoms are all worse at night in bed and by warmth in general, also from the glare of a fire, which is unusually painful, therefore is especially indicated in ciliary blepharitis, caused from working over fires or forges.

Inflammation or blennorrhœa of the lachrymal sac should suggest this remedy, if there is considerable swelling and pain at night, or if the discharge is thin and acrid in nature, providing the general condition of the patient calls for it also.

Ophthalmia neonatorum marked by acrid discharge (usually thin), which makes the cheek sore, and particularly if caused from syphilitic leucorrhœa in the mother, is more quickly relieved by this drug than any other.

In superficial inflammations of the cornea and conjunctiva, either ulcerative, phlyctenular or catarrhal, Mercurius has proved especially serviceable, and we are led to its use by the following symptoms, which have been collected from a great number of cases. In inflammatory conditions dependent upon syphilis, either hereditary or acquired, it is one of the first remedies to be thought of. The ulcers of the cornea are usually quite vascular, though they may be surrounded by a grayish opacity and complicated with existence of pus between the layers of the cornea (onyx). The redness of the conjunctiva is variable, though more frequently of high degree, even in some cases amounting to chemosis. The dread of light is generally very marked, in some cases so intense that they can hardly open the eyes, even in a darkened room, and is more often aggravated from any artificial light, as gaslight, *glare of a fire*, etc. The lachrymation is profuse, *burning* and *excoriating*, and the muco-purulent discharges very *thin and acrid*. The pains are generally severe and vary in character, but are more frequently tearing, burning, shooting or sticking, and are not confined to the eye, but extend up into the forehead and temples; are *always worse at night*, especially before midnight, by heat, damp weather or extreme cold, and are often ameliorated temporarily by cold water. The lids may be spasmodically closed, are thick, red, swollen, even erysipelatously, excoriated by the acrid discharges and sensitive to heat, cold or contact; there is usually biting and burning in the lids, sometimes feels as if there were many fiery points in them, are worse in the open air. The general aggravations in the evening, by gaslight and at night after going to bed, are of the first importance, at the same time the concomitant symptoms of soreness of the head, excoriation of the nose, eruptions on the face, condition of the tongue, offensive breath, night sweats without relief, pain in the bones, especially at night, etc., would lead us in its selection.

Keratitis parenchymatosa which is so often, and according to some authors, always due to hereditary syphilis, very frequently calls for Mercurius, in which affection it has proved extremely valuable.

Kerato-iritis, both with and without hypopion, has been cured with Merc., which would be suggested by the pains and nightly aggravation; in one case in which benefit was derived, the pain was very severe at night, the eye feeling as if it were a ball of fire, the lachrymation was hot and hypopion was present.

In the treatment of episcleritis it should be considered with Thuya, as the following case will illustrate:—A woman, æt. 35, has been troubled for a long time with inflammation of the eyes; the corneæ are covered with scars from old ulcerations; the scleral vessels are injected, especially between the insertion of the recti muscles, where the sclera is slightly bulged and thinned, so that the dark color of the choroid shines through; complains of a steady aching pain in the eye all the time, but worse at night. Merc.^{30} was given, which relieved the pain within a few hours and a rapid recovery ensued.

Mercury has always been and probably always will be the principal remedy for iritis. The solubis has been employed with great success in many cases, though not as commonly useful as the corrosivus. It is especially called for in the syphilitic variety and when condylomata are present in the iris, though its sphere of usefulness is not confined to this form as it is indicated in the rheumatic or any other form of iritis, in mild cases as well as severe, when hypopion is present and when it is absent. The usual symptoms of iritis, contraction, discoloration and immobility of the iris, ciliary injection, haziness of the aqueous, etc., are, of course, found, but the characteristic indications are to be looked for in the pains, which are usually of a tearing, boring character, chiefly around the eye, in the forehead and temples, which are often sore to touch; with this we may have throbbing, shooting and sticking pains in the eye; all of which are always worse at night.

In retinitis or in choroiditis, particularly if dependent upon syphilis, this remedy has been employed with benefit. In these cases the retina is often very sensitive to the glare of a fire. It is the great remedy for diseases of the optic nerve and retina, occurring in workers in founderies.

Gross reports the following case of amblyopia, occurring in a woman, thirty years of age, in which Merc.[12] worked a cure: —For one year her sight had been failing, with frequent temporary loss of vision; even when not using the eyes there are always dark spots or a kind of cloud before the sight, constant lachrymation and aching pressing pain in the eye; cannot bear the light of a fire.

A case of scotoma of the right eye after a fall, with dimness of vision, constant flickering before the eye and floating black specks, is reported cured with Merc.[12].—THORER.

MERCURIUS SUBLIMATUS CORROSIVUS.

Clinical. The corrosive sublimate is more often indicated in severe inflammatory conditions of the eye, especially superficial, than any other form of Mercury.

In certain forms of blepharitis it is frequently very valuable, as in inflammatory swelling of indurated lids, inflammatory swelling of the cheeks and parts around the orbits, which are covered with pustules, or in scrofulous inflammation of the lids, which are red like erysipelas. In these cases the lids are usually *very red and excoriated by the acrid lachrymation, and the pains very severe, particularly at night.*

Merc. corr. is usually more useful in strumous ophthalmia than the solubis, and is chiefly called for if phlyctenules, ulcers or even deep abscesses are found on the cornea, for then the severity of the symptoms would lead us to its selection, as this remedy is especially indicated in the erethistic form of inflammation. The eye is usually very red, and the cornea covered with ulcers and vascular; sometimes it is softened and commences to bulge, and in other cases pannus may be present. *The photophobia is excessive and the lachrymation profuse,* which together with the *ichorous discharges are acrid, excoriating the lids and cheek.* The pains vary in character, though generally very severe and not confined to the eye, but extend into the forehead and temples, and always *worse at night.* The lids are much swollen, erysipelatous, œdematous or indurated, are red and excoriated from the acrid discharges, and are spasmodically closed, rendering it almost impossible to open them, and they often bleed easily upon attempting it. There are also usually present pustules on the cheek around the eye, enlargement of the cervical glands, coated tongue, etc., etc.

Has been employed with benefit in ophthalmia neonatorum, if the discharges are thin and excoriating, and caused from syphilitic leucorrhœa.

For kerato-iritis, it is one of our chief remedies.

In *iritis*, especially the syphilitic variety, it no doubt surpasses any other remedy in frequency of indication, and by some is even considered a specific, providing Atropine is used at the same time locally. The severity of the symptoms and the intensity of the pains at night over the eyes and through them, through the head and in the temples, are our chief indications. The other forms of iritis, as well as the syphilitic, are also often controlled by this drug.

It seems to act beneficially in some cases upon posterior synechiæ, causing them to soften, so that Atropine can tear them, and sometimes even absorbing them entirely, if recent.

Hypopion occurring in the course of abscess of the cornea or iritis, has been frequently quickly absorbed under its use. When the inflammatory process extends to other portions of the uveal tract, particularly if of syphilitic origin, Merc. corr. proves a very valuable remedy.

In retinitis albuminurica, no remedy has been employed with better success in such a large number of cases; the inflammatory process is often seen to rapidly subside, and exudations into the retina disappear under the influence of this remedy. The prescription is chiefly based upon the pathological changes, as the symptoms are so few in the disease.

In superficial inflammations of the eye, Merc. closely resembles several remedies, as Graph., Euphras., Arsen., Sulph., etc., but the severity of the symptoms and nightly aggravation, is much more marked under Merc. than any of the above. Under Graphites the discharges are also acrid and excoriating, and the photophobia often intense, but the pains are not usually so severe as under Merc., and, besides, we usually find the lids cracked, and a moist eruption on the face and behind the ears when Graph. is indicated. The acrid discharges of Euphrasia are generally thick, while those of Mercurius are thin. The character of the pains, general cachexia, etc., will serve to distinguish Arsen. and Sulph.

MEZEREUM.

Muscular twitchings in left upper lid. Aching and tearing in and around the eye, especially in the orbits. Aching around the left eye.

Clinical. In eczematous affections of the lids, face and head, characterized by *thick, hard scabs, from under which pus exudes on pressure*, Mez. is especially useful. It has been given with benefit in blepharitis, pustular conjunctivitis and abscess of the cornea, chiefly when these symptoms have been present.

Ciliary neuralgia, especially after operations upon the eye, has been relieved by this drug.

MURIATIC ACID.

Clinical. The following symptom found in a case of muscular asthenopia, was speedily relieved by Muriatic acid:—Sharp burning pain, extending from the left to the right eye, in the morning, ameliorated by washing.

NATRUM MURIATICUM.

Objective. Spasmodic closure of the lids, especially in the morning. Redness of the white of the eye. Lachrymation acrid, making the canthi sore and red. Lachrymation in the open air (biting).

Subjective. Sensation of sand in the eyes, especially mornings. Aching and itching of the eyes. Smarting pain in the eyes, especially after using. Severe burning of the eyes. Piercing pain above the right eye on looking down, worse evenings.

Vision. Dry burning on writing. *Aching in the eye on looking intently at anything.* Dimness of vision; letters and stitches in sewing run together so they cannot be distinguished. Vision fails on reading. Dark veil passes before the eyes, from right to left, every morning at 10 A.M.

Clinical. Nat. mur. has been successfully employed in a great variety of eye troubles, both superficial and deep.

Is very useful in certain forms of blepharitis, in which the thick inflamed lids smart and burn, with feeling of sand in the eye and acrid lachrymation, which excoriates the lids and cheek, especially if caused from caustics.

Entropion resulting from caustic treatment of granular lids has been cured.

Many cases of stricture of the lachrymal duct, fistula and blennorrhœa of the lachrymal sac, in which the diagnosis cannot be questioned, have been benefited by this remedy.

Hofrichter, in A. H. Z., reports two cases of Morbus Basedowii, characterized by exophthalmus, enlargement of the thyroid gland and palpitation of the heart, causing shortness of breath on the least exertion, which were permanently relieved by Natrum mur.

In pustules and ulcers of the cornea, we frequently derive much benefit from the use of Natrum mur., especially in chronic cases and after the use of caustics, though the symptoms that lead to its selection are not particularly characteristic; thus we have itching and burning in the eyes, and feeling of sand in them, worse in the morning and forenoon; the pains are various, though not severe, except the *sharp pain over the eye on looking down*, which is very marked; the lachrymation is *acrid and excoriating*, making the lids red and sore; the discharges from the eye are also *thin, watery and excoriating* (Merc.); the photophobia is usually marked and the lids spasmodically closed; the skin of the face around the eye, is often found glossy and shining.

A case of ophthalmia blenorrhœa with the following symptoms, was speedily cured:—The lids were very much swollen, of a dark purplish color, and canthi cracked; conjunctiva excessively swollen, chemosed and protruding, upon opening the lids; small points on the upper part of the cornea and profuse muco-purulent discharge; corners of the mouth cracked and sore.

Lorbach reports a case of iritis cured by this remedy.

Hyperæsthesia of the retina has been relieved, in which there has been much lachrymation and burning in the morning, with some conjunctival injection; on looking at a bright light, great photophobia, severe sticking in the temples, and on reading, objects seem to swim before the sight; is especially indicated in chlorotic females.

In asthenopia, particularly muscular, it is one of the most important remedies we possess, especially if there is a *drawing stiff sensation in the muscles of the eyes upon moving them*, with heat and a feeling as though there were a rush of blood to the eyes. The following case will, however, very well illustrate its action:—F. H. G., æt. 28, book-keeper, overstrained his eyes working with various colored inks, writing very fine and often uninterruptedly twelve to fifteen hours; general health good; refraction emmetropic, but considerable weakness of internal recti prevents reading. The eye is hyperæmic, and there is moderate photophobia and constant inclination to close the eyes firmly; touch is unbearable, but hard pressure relieves; sensation as if something sharp and sticking were in the eye. He says, "My eyes itch and burn just like chilblains; I must wipe them often and pull at the lashes." The eyes are very painful on turning them either in or out. Natrum mur.^{200} promptly cured.

Ciliary neuralgia:—Pain in and above the eye (especially right) coming on and going off with the sun; eye congested, sore and painful when moved; can bear neither natural nor artificial light; pain from lamplight; could not hurt more if the eye were pulled from the socket; discouraged; craves salt. Two cases cured by C. M. Chamberlain.

Tülf recommends this remedy, and has used it with benefit in "amblyopia and amaurosis," with congestion or inflammation of the eye, with pressing, boring, sticking and burning pains, if dependent upon some menstrual disorder, especially in chlorotic females, in whom headache, vertigo, sadness, etc., in the morning precede the menstrual flow.

NATRUM SULPHURICUM.

Crawling sensation in the eyes. Great dryness and burning of the eyes; grows worse from afternoon to evening; it seemed as if her eyeballs were hot.

Clinical. Has been found of use in conjunctivitis granulosa, in which the granulations appear like small blisters (Thuya).—GRAUVOGL.

As a local application to maculæ corneæ, it has been of excellent service.

NITRIC ACID.

Objective. Swelling of the lids. Small wart on upper lid. Inflammation of conjunctiva. Lachrymation and agglutination of the eyes.

Subjective. Burning in the lids mornings. Aching in the eyes, stinging and matterating. Stitches in the eyes. Photophobia.

Clinical. Nitric acid is of especial importance in diseases of the eye of a syphilitic origin, or if resulting from the abuse of potash or mercury.

The following case shows its importance in tumors of the lid:—A woman, æt. 28, had on the right lower lid a large condyloma, which was suppurating and bled easily when touched; it seemed to arise from a lens shaped body on the inner surface of the lower lid; ectropion had commenced; the eye and vicinity were much inflamed, with burning, sticking pain, profuse hot lachrymation and agglutination mornings. Thuya[6] was of little service, but Nitric acid[6] cured.—Wähle.

In scrofulous ophthalmia it has proved of value (according to Goullon and Dudgeon), if the lids are much inflamed and swollen, and there is intense photophobia, excessive lachrymation and great redness.

Much benefit has been derived from the use of this remedy in gonorrhœal ophthalmia, as the following will illustrate:—A young man, æt. 19, had been troubled three days with a severe ophthalmia of the right eye, arising from gonorrhœal contagion; both lids were very much swollen, red, hard and painful, so that it was with difficulty that the ball could be seen; conjunctiva very hyperæmic and chemosed, with pressing out pain in the eye; cornea dim, great photophobia, constant lachrymation and copious secretion of yellow pus, which flows down the cheek; there was burning pain in the eye, moderate by day, but increased at night; the cheek around the eye was also much swollen and painful. The local application of a solution of Nitric acid, immediately relieved the pain and soon cured.—Knorre.

Ulcers and maculæ of the cornea are said to have been removed.

Irritating flow of tears after traumatic injury of the eye, was relieved.—H. Goullon.

Berridge reports a case of syphilitic iritis, cured with Nitric acid[200]:—On lying down or even inclining the head from the upright position, feeling as if warm water were flowing over and from both eyes, first right, then left. Ameliorated by cold water.

NUX VOMICA.

Objective. Twitching of the lids. Inflammation of the eyes. Blood exudes from the eye. Lachrymation.

Subjective. The margin of the lid pains as if rubbed sore, especially mornings and on touch. Biting in the eyes, especially in the external canthus as from salt, with lachrymation.

Photophobia (cannot bear daylight) mornings, with obscuration of sight.

Clinical. The power of Nux vom. to relieve nervous irritability, has led to its beneficial use in diverse affections of the eye, as the following clinical record will show.

In ciliary blepharitis, with smarting and dryness of the lids, *especially in the morning*, our remedy will be found in Nux vom. It is also indicated in ciliary blepharitis dependent upon certain forms of gastric disturbance.

From its action in spasmodic affections, we are led to its use in blepharospasmus, in which it has been given with benefit, though not so frequently indicated as Agaricus.

As a remedy for conjunctivitis it is not as often called for as when the cornea becomes involved, though in both catarrhal and scrofulous inflammation of the conjunctiva benefit has been derived, especially if there is marked morning aggravation and the usual concomitant symptoms.

Both Hartman and Altschul recommend its use very highly, from experience, in conjunctivitis, in which there is great tendency to hemorrhage, so that not only ecchymosed spots are found in the conjunctival tissue, but blood oozes out between the lids. Even in spontaneous hemorrhage from the conjunctiva it has proved useful, as might be expected from its symptomatology.

Good results have been obtained from its use in ophthalmia neonatorum, in which the lids are much swollen, bleed easily and the child is troubled with vomiting, constipation and flatulent colic.

Old cases of trachoma, especially if complicated with pannus, that have had much treatment, are often benefited by this remedy. It is, however, frequently of use, either to commence the treatment or as an intercurrent remedy in trachoma, with or without pannus, though it rarely effects a cure unassisted by any other drug.

It is frequently indicated in ulcers and pustules of the cornea, especially the former, *with excessive photophobia.* An important point regarding the photophobia, as well as the other symptoms, is the *morning aggravation*, which is rarely absent. In addition to this, we usually have much lachrymation and a variety of pains, none of which, however, can be said to be very characteristic, though the following are a few which have been relieved: sharp, darting pains in the eye and over it, in some cases extending to the top of the head and always worse in the morning; burning pain in the eyes and lids; tearing pain in the eye at night, awakening from sleep; eye feels pressed out, whenever she combs her hair; sensation of hot water in the eye; pain in the lower lid as if something were cutting it. Sometimes relief from the pain is obtained by bathing the eyes in cold water. Cases that have been overdosed by external and internal medication are particularly adapted to this remedy.

Has proved useful in iritis, as in one case of the syphilitic variety, with moderate ciliary injection, some photophobia, hot lachrymation, worse in the morning, and great sensitiveness to the air, though it cannot be often indicated.

Its action upon the muscles should not be overlooked, for though it is not often called for in strabismus, still it has benefited some cases, periodic in character, especially aggravated by mental excitement or when caused by an injury.

For paralytic affections of the muscles it may be sometimes useful, as in one case of paresis of the internal rectus with diplopia, always worse from the use of stimulants or tobacco.

Hyperæsthesia of the retina, with frequent pains to the top of the head, sleepless nights and awakening cross in the morning, was promptly relieved by Nux vom.

Even after the deeper structures have become inflamed, benefit has been derived, as in a case of chorio-retinitis, with much throbbing pain, especially in the left eye and worse in the morning, ball sore to touch, upper part of the sclera bright red, burning pain in the eye not relieved by bathing, and aggravation of the symptoms on lying down.

In choroiditis disseminata it is a prominent remedy, especially if occurring in persons addicted to the use of stimulants; its special indications do not vary from those already given in speaking of other diseases.

Four cases of "arthritic ophthalmia" (glaucoma?), occurring in old persons, with tearing pains in the orbit, borders of lids red and very sensitive to touch, great photophobia on awaking in the morning and much lachrymation, are reported cured.

Of late years strychnia has been employed very extensively by the old school in the treatment of atrophy of the optic nerve and various forms of amblyopia. It is used chiefly by hypodermic injection and in many cases with marked success. We also often find Nux vom. useful in atrophy of the optic nerve, checking the progress of the disease and in many cases restoring the vision to a limited extent, though it is, of course, impossible to restore the sight wholly, if genuine atrophy has once commenced.

In amblyopia potatorum or impairment of vision, due chiefly to the use of intoxicating drinks or even to dissipation in general, no remedy will more frequently restore to power the function of the benumbed nerve.

Dr. Woodyatt says in U. S. M. and S. J.:—"In various forms of trouble I have been led to give Nux vom. for a blurring of sight by over-heating and nearly every time with benefit."

OPIUM.

Clinical. The use of this drug in ophthalmology has been very limited, except as an anodyne.

We, however, have two very interesting cases in which Opium rapidly cured:—A woman, æt. 35, had been troubled with her eyes for six weeks. Upon examination, total paralysis of the accommodation, with impaired sensibility of the retina of the right eye, and partial paralysis of the accommodation of the left eye was found. It was supposed to be due to the use of a cosmetic, which probably contained carbonate of lead. The other symptoms present were as follows: almost constantly frontal headache, vertigo, with darting pains from the occiput to the forehead, distressing feeling of emptiness in the stomach, especially in the morning, bowels constipated, and a sensation of pain and constriction as of a band encircling her chest in the line of the pleura. Nux vom.[2] failed. Opium[3] cured.—W. A. PHILLIPS.

The second case was one of embolism of the central artery of the retina; the arteries were bloodless, veins engorged and stagnant, and hemorrhagic spots on the disk. Came on after a severe attack of neuralgia. The face was very red, numb and drawn to the right side, tongue protruded to the right side, speech was imperfect, nearly voiceless, except with effort, and pain in the back. All the pains were on the right side. Under the use of Opium, alone, he gradually recovered not only his vision, but also power over the paralyzed parts.

PARIS QUADRIFOLIA.

Clinical. This drug produced a permanent cure of paralysis of the iris and ciliary muscle, supposed to be due to an injury received two years previous; there was pain drawing from the eye to the back of the head, where there was a sore spot, even pressure with the finger would cause her to cry out; many black floating specks before the vision were present.

The following symptoms have also been relieved by Paris:—*Pain in the eyes, as if pulled into the head.* Double vision. Headache worse in the evening, with confusion of the whole forehead and sensation as if skin of the forehead were drawn together and the bones scraped sore, with inflamed lids, red margins and sensation *as if threads drew from the eye into the middle of the head.* Tension around the brow, as though the skin were thick and difficult to wrinkle.

PETROLEUM.

Aching in the eyes severe, worse evenings by the light. Itching and sticking in the eyes. Burning and aching, and obscuration on exerting the vision. Cannot open the eyes mornings; sight is dim and misty.

Clinical. Within the last few years the purified preparations of petroleum, cosmoline, vaseline, etc., have been used to a great extent and with much benefit as external applications in cases of blepharitis; in fact we know of no better external remedy for this affection; it prevents the formation of new scabs and the agglutination of the lids, besides seeming to exert a beneficial influence over the progress of the disease. At the same time the use of Petrol. internally is highly recommended, especially if connected with the characteristic occipital headache, rough skin, etc. Cases in which ciliary blepharitis has resulted from conjunctivitis granulosa, also when it has been a sequela of small-pox, with smarting and sticking-like pains in the inner canthus, have been cured by this drug.

In disorders of the lachrymal apparatus, especially blennorrhœa of the lachrymal sac, this remedy is of the first importance, though its choice depends chiefly upon the concomitant symptoms.

Lachrymal fistulæ are reported cured, which may be the case if of very recent origin.

Benefit has been gained from its use in conjunctivitis granulosa, though it is not frequently called for, except in some cases complicated with pannus; for in the latter affection, especially if found in a scrofulous habit with considerable white discharge from the eye, roughness of the cheek, etc., we find a valuable remedy in Petrol.

Scrofulous ophthalmia with pains at the root of the nose, swelling of the lids and purulent discharge from the eyes and nostrils, also pustular conjunctivitis with considerable inflammation of the lids, has been cured.

Iritis, especially the syphilitic variety, with dull pulsating pain in the occiput, occasionally calls for Petrol.

PHELLANDRIUM.

Clinical. The following case is reported cured in the Brit. Jour. of Hom.:—Ciliary neuralgia, great pain on attempting to read or sew, fearful intolerance of light, must sit in a dark corner, lids swollen and half closed, conjunctiva of lid and caruncle inflamed, red scarlet, headache like a heavy weight on the top of the head, with burning and shooting pains in the temples.

PHOSPHORUS.

Choroid hyperæmic and musci volitantes. Balls pain as if compressed, aggravated on looking. Aching and heaviness in the eyes, like sleepiness.

Vision. Vision fails on reading. On reading (either by day or candle-light) the eye pains. Myopia, outlines of distant objects blurred. Vision better mornings in twilight. Sees objects best near, at a distance everything is seen as through smoke or gauze; even near objects cannot be distinctly seen long; vision better if the pupil is dilated by shading the eyes with the hands. Dark bodies and spots before the eyes. Black points float across vision. Sparks before the eyes in dusk. Green halo around candle-light evenings. Objects seen as through a gauze. Amblyopia.

Clinical. In external affections of the eye very little benefit has been derived from the use of Phosphorus, although Berridge reports one case of a white pustule (?) on the outer segment of the left cornea, cured by a high potency of this remedy.

Its greatest sphere of action is to be found in diseases of the fundus, especially in disturbance of function of the optic nerve, though its action upon the muscles of the eye cannot be ignored.

Paralysis of the muscles, particularly if accompanied by spermatorrhœa, sexual abuse, hemorrl oids, etc., are especially adapted to Phos., according to Tavignot, who relates two interesting cases in which it proved useful. One was a case of total paralysis of the third pair of nerves, ptosis, eye turned outwards, mydriasis, etc., occurring in a woman. Electricity was of no avail, but under the use of Phos. she entirely recovered. The other was a case of paralysis of the sixth pair of nerves, accompanied by spermatorrhœa, resulting from onanism.

Not only in paralysis, but also in weakness of the internal recti muscles has this drug been found indicated, as in a case of asthenopia muscularis, in which there was pain and stiffness of the eyeballs on moving them, and at times a feeling of heat in the eyes as after looking at a fire.

The following instructive case, reported by Dr. Hall, in H. M., shows the power of this remedy in asthenopia:—A woman, æt. 21, had been troubled some time with a blurring of vision, which came on suddenly after reading. Since then has had a dull pain in the eye after reading a short time, compelling her to desist. At times her sight is very dim and black spots pass before the eyes. Is always worse from looking at any bright, shining object, and in the lamplight, but is better in the twilight, which is the best time of day for her. The lids feel heavy in the morning. Phos. worked a brilliant cure.

Benefit has been seen from its use in stopping the progress of cataract.

In both hyperæmia and inflammation of the retina, good results have been obtained. In one case it relieved very quickly a congestion of the retina, in which the balls were sore on motion, no photophobia, pains extending from the eyes to the top of the head.

Is indicated in various forms of retinitis, as one would be led to suppose from its symptomatology, but especially in that rare form retinitis nyctalopia. From its pathogenesis, we are also led to believe that it will prove a valuable addition to our list of remedies for retinitis albuminurica, and some experience seems to corroborate this view.

In both disseminate and serous choroiditis, relief has been found from the use of Phos. In the various diseases of the fundus in which it is called for, there will usually be found photopsies or chromopsies (in one case of choroiditis disseminata, the latter were red in color). Rapidly increasing myopia has been checked in its progress.

The following symptoms observed in an excessively hypermetropic person, were quickly relieved:—Mistiness before the vision, with attacks of vanishing of sight; eyes weak so must close them; balls seem large and difficult to get the lids over them; lids agglutinated.

The cases of so-called amaurosis, are many in which the sight has been restored by Phosphorus, and even in the genuine amaurosis, "where the patient sees nothing and the doctor also nothing," much has been gained by its use. That form of amaurosis consequent upon sexual excesses, especially call for this remedy, while other forms for which no cause could be discovered, have been greatly benefited.

PHYSOSTIGMA VENOSA.

Clinical. Calabar bean applied locally to the eye, produces at first slight twitching of the lids, soon followed by contraction of the pupil and spasm of the ciliary muscle, from its action as an irritant to the oculo-motor nerve. In this respect antagonistic to Atropine, which causes dilatation of the pupil and paralysis of the ciliary muscle, by paralyzing the filaments of the third pair.

For this reason it has often been employed as a mechanical agent in overcoming the temporary ill effects of Atropine, when used for purposes of examination, etc. Its action, however, is so short that it requires frequent instillation to overcome them thoroughly.

It has also been used as a mechanical aid in tearing away adhesions of the iris, especially to the cornea, and in cases of deep ulceration of the cornea when at the periphery, so that if perforation occurs, the pupillary edge of the iris will not be drawn into the opening.

Has also been of service, used locally, in paralysis of the accommodation and dilatation of the pupil, consequent upon loss of power of the oculo-motor nerve.

Its usefulness is not confined to its mechanical power, for when given internally upon physiological principles and according to the law of "similia," it is valuable.

Twitching of the lid should direct our attention to this drug, especially if combined with spasm of the ciliary muscle, as in one case in which there was twitching around the eyes, patient cannot read at all without much pain, frontal headache aggravated by any light. Physostig. gave quick relief.

Dr. Woodyatt adopting the theory that myopia in a great majority of cases, is due to spasm of the ciliary muscle, or, at least, that its increase depends upon this cause, has given Physostigma, 2d dec., in several cases with excellent results, often reducing the degree of myopia very perceptibly, and even in some cases restoring the vision entirely. The symptoms of irritation, pain after using eyes, musci volitantes, flashes of light, etc., which might lead us to suspect spasm of the accommodation, are usually present and are soon relieved, while in other cases no symptoms of irritation were to be perceived, still the administration of Physostigma was followed by favorable results.

Prominent oculists of the old school are employing it locally in muscular asthenopia, with benefit. A weak solution is instilled into the eyes, once or twice a day, for weeks.

PHYTOLACCA DECANDRA.

Clinical. Has been employed with some success in ameliorating, if not curing malignant ulcers of the lid, as lupus, epithelioma, etc.

A very interesting case of suppurative choroiditis (panophthalmitis) in the right eye of a child, after a needle operation for cataract, occurred in Dr. Liebold's clinic:—The lids were enormously swollen, very hard and red, conjunctiva chemosed, anterior chamber filled with pus, and cornea tending towards suppuration; child pale, weak and restless. Phytolacca externally and internally was given with marked relief, the inflammatory symptoms rapidly subsiding under its employment. (Compare with Rhus.)

PLUMBUM METALLICUM.

Clinical. Theuerkauf reports the following case occurring in a woman:—Hypopion following iritis, which filled one-half of the anterior chamber; tearing pains at night in the eye and forehead, which prevented her from sleeping; vision was so poor, she could hardly distinguish night from day. Plumbum[15] cured.

PRUNUS SPINOSA.

Clinical. As a remedy for ciliary neuralgia, whether originating from some diseased condition of the eye or not, there are few, if any drugs more often called for than Prunus.

The character of the pains furnish our chief indications; thus we have pain in the eyeball, as if it were crushed or wrenched, or *pain as if pressed asunder;* again we often find the pain of a *sharp, shooting* character, extending through the eye back into the brain, or this sharp pain may be seated above the eye, extending into and around it, or over the corresponding side of the head. Sometimes the pain will commence behind the ears and shoot forward to the eye, but, as already remarked, is generally of this sharp, piercing character. Motion usually aggravates and rest relieves the severity of the pains.

These pains to which Prunus is adapted, are especially found in disorders of the internal structures of the eye, therefore it has been given in many of these cases and with marked benefit. Particularly in sclerotico-choroiditis post. have good results been obtained in stopping the progress of the disease.

Dr. O'Connor, who first brought this drug into notice in ophthalmic affections, says he has used it with benefit in the following cases:—"Two cases of chorio-retinitis in myopic patients, with sclerectasia posterior and fluidity of the vitreous, with floating opacities in it (hemorrhagic). One case of irido-choroiditis, no fluidity of the vitreous and no floating opacities. Another case of irido-cyclitis with anterior synechiæ, and also once in an old lady, æt. 76, who had paralysis of the right side and cornea nearly opaque, with excessive congestion of the superficial and deep vessels of the conjunctiva and sclerotic." In all these cases the pains were the chief indications.

Other cases of choroiditis, either with or without retinal complication, have been quickly relieved and the vision restored, so far as possible, in the degenerated condition of the tissues.

The opacities and haziness of the vitreous, occurring during the course of choroideal troubles, have been seen to disappear under Prunus, when given in accordance with the usual indications.

PSORINUM.

Clinical. As one of our anti-psorics, this remedy occupies an important position in the treatment of many ophthalmic disorders, dependent upon scrofula, etc.

Ciliary blepharitis, especially if of a chronic recurrent nature, is often amenable to this drug; they are usually old chronic cases, with no marked local symptoms to govern us in the selection of the remedy. Inflammation of the lids of a more acute character, as when the internal surface has become much congested and combined with great photophobia, so that the child cannot open the eyes but lies constantly on the face, has been cured.

In old recurrent cases of pustular inflammation of the cornea and conjunctiva, most benefit seems to have been gained. The chronic nature, recurrent form and scrofulous basis, are our chief indications.

Bærtl reports a case of "pterygium" terminating in an ulcer at the margin of the cornea, with dry itching eruption on the palms of the hands, cured by Psor.[6]

A case of serous choroiditis occurring in a young lady, about 21, was greatly improved under its use; there was some ciliary congestion and great haziness of the vitreous, so that the optic nerve was only discerned with great difficulty, and then was found decidedly hyperæmic, as was the whole fundus. Some headache was present, especially in the morning; also a profuse sweat of the palms of the hands all the time.

PULSATILLA.

Objective. Margin of lower lid inflamed and swollen, with lachrymation mornings. Lids swollen and red. *Stye* on the lid and inflammation of the white of the eye, now in one, now in other canthus, with drawing, tensive pain therein on moving muscles of face, and with ulcerated nostrils. Twitching of lids. A red spot in the white of the eye near the cornea. Lachrymation, especially in the open, cold air.

Subjective. Itching of the ball in the external canthus evenings, and agglutination mornings. Sticking and pressive pains in the eye. Aching in the eye on reading. Burning and itching in the eyes, must scratch and rub them, especially evenings.

Vision. Diplopia. Obscuration of vision, with nausea and pale face. Obscuration of vision transient. Fiery circles constantly widen and become worse toward noon, better toward evening.

Clinical. This remedy is very frequently indicated in a great variety of diseases of the eye, but in its selection we are governed in a great measure by the temperament and general symptoms of the patient. Those eye troubles, especially the superficial found in the negro race, as well as those occurring in the mild, tearful female, seem to be particularly benefited by Pulsatilla.

For blepharitis, both acute and chronic, it is a valuable remedy, especially if there is inflammation of the glands of the lids, both meibomian and sebaceous (blepharo-adenitis); also in cases of blepharitis in which there is a great tendency to the formation of styes or abscesses on the margin of the lids; often called for in blepharitis resulting from indulgence in high living or fat food, and if accompanied by acne of the face. The swelling and redness of the lids vary in different instances, as does also the discharge, though more frequently we find profuse secretion from the meibomian glands causing agglutination of the lids in the morning. The sensations experienced are usually of an itching, burning character and are aggravated in the evening, in a warm room, or in a cold draught of air, but ameliorated in the cool open air.

As a remedy for styes (Hordeola) it has no equal, and by some is even considered almost specific, as in a great majority of cases it will cause them to abort before the formation of pus has taken place.

In tarsal tumors, especially of recent origin, subject to inflammation or when accompanied by a catarrhal condition of the eye, help has been derived from its use.

Spasmodic action of the lids, with lachrymation and photophobia, has been relieved.

Its action upon the lachrymal sac is very decided, and it has proved a valuable remedy in blennorhœa, in which the discharge is very profuse and bland, especially when occurring in a Pulsatilla temperament.

Dacryocystitis may, sometimes, be checked at its commencement with this drug, though it is also useful during the whole course of the disease.

Pulsatilla has been successfully employed in a great variety of conjunctival and corneal affections, as in simple catarrhal conjunctivitis, especially the acute form (though also useful in the chronic) either resulting from a cold, an attack of measles or other cause, and when there is present a variable amount of redness, even in some cases chemosis, burning, itching or sticking in the eye, usually worse in the evening, when out in the wind and after reading, but relieved in the cool open air; the lachrymation is often profuse by day and purulent at night, though generally a moderately profuse muco-purulent discharge of a whitish color and bland character, which agglutinates the lids in the morning, is to be found. Catarrhal ophthalmia observed during an attack of measles; catarrhal ophthalmia with gastric bilious symptoms or inflammation of the eyes consequent upon traumatic causes, have been benefited by Puls.

In purulent ophthalmia we frequently find Puls. of use, especially if the discharge is profuse and bland, and the concomitant symptoms also indicate its selection.

That form of blennorrhœa of the conjunctiva, caused from the gonorrhœal contagion, has been reported cured.

Another frequent form of purulent ophthalmia, found in newborn children (ophthalmia neonatorum) has been greatly benefited, even in some instances well marked cases have been cured without the use of any other drug. It seems, however, especially useful in this trouble as an intercurrent remedy during the treatment by Argentum Nitricum, for often when the improvement is at a stand-still, a few doses of Pulsatilla will materially hasten the progress of the cure.

Has been employed with some success in trachoma, usually uncomplicated with pannus. The granulations are generally very fine and eye sometimes dry, or may be accompanied by excessive secretion of bland mucus. There may also be soreness of the ball to touch and itching, or pain in the eye, worse in the evening and better in the cool air, or by cold applications. Especially adapted to cases occurring in anæmic amenorrhœic females.

Another large class of superficial ophthalmic disorders in which Puls. is particularly useful, is to be found in scrofulous ophthalmia or phlyctenular keratitis and conjunctivitis. Here it has proved one of our sheet anchors in the treatment, especially if the pustules are on the conjunctiva. The dread of light is often absent and usually moderate in degree. The lachrymation is not acrid but more abundant in the open air, while the other discharges are generally profuse, thick, white or yellow, and bland. The pains are more often of a pressing, stinging character though they vary greatly. The lids may be swollen but are not excoriated, though *subject to styes.* The eyes feel worse on getting warm from exercise or in a warm room and generally in the evening, but are ameliorated in the open air and by cold applications. The concomitant symptoms of ear disorders, thirstlessness, gastric derangement, amenorrhoea, etc., must be taken into consideration.

Has been successfully given in ulcers of the cornea, especially if superficial, and resulting from phlyctenules. Of late we have observed excellent results from the use of Pulsatilla in those small ulcers which prove so intractable to treatment, occurring near the centre of the cornea with no vascular supply, especially if found in strumous subjects, with phlyctenules on the cornea or conjunctiva; considerable photophobia and pain.

A case of episcleritis circumscribed, situated between the superior and external recti muscles, was very promptly relieved by this remedy. It occurred in a man, highly myopic; the sclera was slightly bulged, and some itching, sticking pain in the ball, with dimness of vision. His eyes always felt much better in the open air.

Benefit has been observed from its use in iritis, with dry, burning heat in and about the eye, œdema of the lid, secretion of mucus, etc., though it will rarely be called for in this affection.

Bojanus, in A. H. Z., 80, reports a very interesting case of hyperæmia of the retina, occurring after suppression of acne of the face, in a woman, æt. 32. She sees as through a veil and mostly double; reading is difficult; worse by candlelight; after exerting the eyes, she has a pain in the right side of the head and ringing in the right ear; her menses often omit for a whole term, are very scanty, of too short duration, and attended with excruciating, colicky pains, and bearing down; appetite and sleep are good; bowels constipated; ophthalmoscopic examination shows great hyperæmia of the retina; injection of the central vessels and varicosity of the veins. She is of a good natured, yielding, tearful disposition. Puls.^{200}, with an occasional dose of Sulphur 30 or 200, cured the case.

Its influence upon choroidal affections has been proven, as in a case of hyperæmia of the choroid, consequent upon hyperopia; cannot look long at any object; subject to severe neuralgic headaches extending into the eyes; head feels full and congested; is a great tea drinker. Puls. effected a cure.

Payr recommends this drug in sub-acute cases of choroiditis in persons subject to arthritis vaga, venous hyperæmia of the capillaries, pressing, tearing and throbbing pain in the head, with heaviness and vertigo, dull sight, photophobia and fiery circles before the eyes. Female individuals, with mild and yielding disposition, scanty and delayed menstruation.

H. Robinson reports the following symptom cured, which is not rarely observed in inflammations of the fundus:—Cloudiness of vision, with a kind of flashing of fire, as though she had received a slap in the face.

Asthenopia accommodativa, with much aching sensation in the eyes after using; also darting pains in the eyes after sewing, in asthenopia from general prostration, have been cured.

A case of hemeralopia with amenorrhœa, was cured with Puls. tinct.—BETHMANN.

RANUNCULUS BULBOSUS.

Clinical. We found this remedy indicated in one case of herpes zoster supra-orbitalis, with bluish black vescicles, high fever and the usual pains accompanying this disease. The success, consequent upon the use of the drug, was exceedingly brilliant.

Has been used by Billig in two cases of hemeralopia:—A woman, thirty years of age, became night-blind during the seventh month of her pregnancy; there was heat, biting and pressure in the eyes; lids and conjunctiva slightly red, with lachrymation and a little pus in the angles of the eye; dull appearance of the eyes with dilated pupils. Ranunculus[1] cured. A son of the above, æt. 4, also became suddenly night-blind; only slight dilatation of the pupil was present in this case. Ranunculus[1] also relieved.

RATANHIA.

Clinical. Pterygium has been put on record as cured by this drug, in the first or second potency, by Hughes and by Newton.

RHODODENDRON.

Clinical. In insufficiency of the internal recti muscles, (asthenopia muscularis) benefit has been derived, as was well marked in a case in which darting pains like arrows through the eye from the head, always worse before a storm, was an accompanying symptom; also in a case reported by Berridge, in which very hot lachrymation from the right eye occurred upon staring or writing.

Very marked and satisfactory results were obtained from Rhod. in the following case:—A man, about forty, complained of gradual failure of sight, accompanied by periodically recurring pains of the most violent character, involving the eyeball, extending to orbit and head, always worse at the approach of a storm, and ameliorated when the storm broke out. The patient had a strongly marked rheumatic diathesis and general good health. On examination the pupils were noticed to be somewhat dilated and sluggish. T + 1 in both eyes. Pulsation of the retinal veins, but no excavation of the optic nerve. Field of vision not circumscribed. Hm. $\frac{1}{30}$. Vision improved by glasses, but could not be brought above $\frac{20}{30}$. The ability to use the eye was greatly relieved by convex 36, and afterward by convex 24, but the attacks of pain continued to recur and his vision suffered sensible impairment from every attack of pain. These were promptly relieved after Rhod., so that within six months he was entirely relieved of the attacks, though he has continued to keep the medicine by him for several years. His vision has gradually improved so that it is now fully $\frac{20}{30}$.

RHUS TOXICODENDRON.

Objective. Inflammation of the lids. The upper lid seems swollen and aches, ameliorated in the open air. A hard, red swelling on left lower lid near internal canthus, like a stye, with pressive pains. Eyes closed by the *great swelling of the* *lids*, and are inflamed. Eyes red and agglutinated mornings. *Lachrymation.*

Subjective. Drawing and tearing in the eyebrow and malar bones. Biting, itching in right upper lid, ameliorated by rubbing. Aching pain in the ball on turning it or pressing on it. Evenings about eight, a heaviness and stiffness in the lids as if paralyzed, as if too heavy to move.

Clinical. The clinical application of this drug is extensive in ophthalmic disorders, and merits careful consideration. It is of value in many troubles, as will be shown hereafter, but it seems especially adapted to the severer forms of the inflammatory process, in which there is a great tendency to suppuration or even when the formation of pus has already taken place.

It will be seen from a study of the symptoms which Rhus produces upon the palpebræ, that its curative power is chiefly exerted upon those symptoms of the lids which are dependent upon inflammation of the deeper structures. Although we may often find it a valuable remedy in uncomplicated blepharitis, especially of the acute form, as when there is a tendency to the formation of an abscess, and the lids are œdematously swollen, accompanied by profuse lachrymation and pains, which are worse at night, and relieved by warm application.

We also occasionally find it useful in chronic inflammation of the lids, in which there is puffiness of the lids and face, enlargement of the meibomian glands, falling out of the ciliæ, itching and biting in the lids, sensation of dryness of the eyes and burning in the internal canthus, with acrid lachrymation in the morning and in the open air, or as is more commonly the case, constant profuse lachrymation, which may be acrid or not.

Simple œdema of the lids has been relieved.

In erysipelas of the lids it is very important, whether of traumatic origin or not, if there is œdematous erysipelatous swelling of the lids and face, with small watery vesicles scattered over the surface, and drawing pains in the cheek and head.

In any of these cases in which the lids are affected, there is frequently spasmodic closure, with profuse lachrymation upon opening them, which more than ever points to the employment of Rhus.

Ptosis has been relieved under this remedy; it is probably adapted to that variety caused from exposure to cold or *wet* (Caust.).

For orbital cellulitis it is a remedy of the first importance, and will no doubt be oftener called for than any other drug, whatever may be the origin of the trouble, whether traumatic or not, as the picture of the disease corresponds very closely to the symptomatology of the drug, and experience has proven the truth of the assertion, that it is *the* remedy in the treatment of this dangerous malady. Some alarming cases of this disease occurring in our own experience, have been promptly arrested by this drug. In one case one eye was entirely lost, and had been operated upon with a view of providing free exit for the suppurative process, and the disease was making alarming and rapid progress in the other eye. Rhus[1] speedily arrested its progress.

In paresis or paralysis of any of the muscles of the eyeball, resulting from rheumatism, exposure to cold, getting the feet wet, etc., this remedy is very useful, and should be compared with Causticum in frequency of indication.

Simple conjunctivitis caused from exposure to wet (Calc.) frequently calls for Rhus, especially if the conjunctiva is much chemosed, with some photophobia, profuse lachrymation, and œdematous swelling of the lids.

In severe cases of conjunctivitis granulosa with pannus, the intensity of the symptoms may occasionally be relieved by the use of this remedy, and possibly a cure be effected.

In ophthalmia neonatorum it has been very highly recommended by Hartman, Garay and others, and it will probably be frequently found of great service in this disorder, when the lids are red, œdematously swollen and spasmodically closed. The palpebral conjunctiva is especially inflamed, and when the lids are opened, a thick red swelling appears, with thick, yellow, purulent discharge; the child is also usually cachectic, restless and head hot. It has been used both externally and internally with advantage, and should prove a valuable remedy for this trouble.

In ulcers and pustules of the cornea, Rhus has been often employed with success, especially in the latter and superficial forms of ulceration, in which the photophobia is very great so that the patient lies constantly on the face, the lachrymation very profuse, so that the tears gush out on opening the spasmodically closed lids (which are also usually much swollen, especially the upper) and the conjunctiva quite red even to chemosis. The skin of the face around the eye is often covered with a Rhus eruption; and the remedy is, of course, especially suitable to persons of a rheumatic diathesis. The symptoms are usually worse at night, after midnight and in damp weather, therefore the patients are restless at night and disturbed by bad dreams.

Its action, however, is not confined to the superficial variety of keratitis, as great benefit has been observed from its use in suppuration of the cornea, especially if consequent upon cataract extraction.

Stens, Sr., in A. H. Z., reports the following case of opacity of the cornea:—"Patient, æt. 45, totally blind. The cornea is filled between its lamellæ with a thick whitish exudation; the iris is distorted. Eye doctors have made iridectomy; no sight. The cause of the blindness must therefore have had a deeper seat. Patient has in former years been subject to erysipelas of the face. Cold water applications had suppressed the eruption. Since then he began to complain of weak vision, which gradually grew to total blindness. Rhus tox.[1], night and morning, restored him to sight."

Several cases of kerato-iritis have been reported cured by Schelling, Segin and others. The following case described by Segin, well illustrates the class of cases to which Rhus is adapted:—A woman, about thirty, was troubled with severe pain in the right eyeball and great sensitiveness, so could not bear the slightest touch or the least exposure to light; the cornea was dull, sclerotic injected, iris discolored and sluggish;

there was an eruption of small red pimples around the eye, and severe burning, tearing pain in the neighborhood of the eye, worse in the morning and at night, so could not sleep. Rhus[5] cured. In another case reported by Schelling, which resulted from cessation of the menses, and was followed by an attack of furuncles, eruption on the head, etc., the pains were of a tearing, sticking character in both temples and forehead, extending deep into the head; also pressure deep in orbits, burning in the eyes, etc. Rhus[200] relieved.

In simple idiopathic or rheumatic iritis, this drug has proved serviceable, especially in those cases resulting from exposure to wet or if the predisposing cause can be referred to a rheumatic diathesis.

Its grandest sphere of action is to be found in suppurative iritis or in the still more severe cases in which the inflammatory process has involved the remainder of the uveal tract (ciliary body and choroid), especially if of traumatic origin, as after cataract extraction. As a remedy in this dangerous form of inflammation of the eye, it stands unrivalled, no other drug having as yet, been found equal to it in importance in this serious malady. The symptoms of the drug will be seen to correspond very closely to a great majority of the cases. The lids are red, swollen and œdematous, especially the upper, and spasmodically closed with profuse gushes of hot tears upon opening them; sac-like swelling of the conjunctiva, and yellow purulent, mucous discharge; pain in and around the eye; swelling of the cheek and surrounding parts, besides the usual concomitant symptoms. For suppurative inflammation of a part or whole of the uveal tract of non-traumatic origin, and even if the formation of pus has already taken place, Rhus has been known to cause its absorption and restore the eye "ad integrum." We also think from experience, that it serves to a certain extent to prevent suppurative inflammation after severe operations upon the eye, though do not by any means consider it a sure preventative.*

* If most prompt results are not found from the higher potencies in a few hours, the first should be resorted to. This is a most important note to make, for not a moment can be lost in arresting the disease, nor can we afford to produce an aggravation in a sensitive subject with large doses.

In Rückert's suppl. vol., sixteen cases diagnosticated "arthritic ophthalmia," are reported cured. A part of them were found in old gouty subjects, and the remainder proceeded from a cold, caused by working in water. There was tearing pain in the eyes, especially at night; the pain was increased by any movement of the eye and extended into the brain; the borders of the lids pain as if ulcerated, and are sensitive to touch; constant lachrymation; painful stiffness of the neck.

Rhus radicans has been often employed with great success in scrofulous ophthalmia, in which the same symptoms are present which have been given under Rhus tox.

RUTA GRAVEOLENS.

Twitching observable in the muscles of the brow.

Weak pressive pain in the right eye, with obscuration as if one had looked too long at trying objects. Heat and fire in the eyes, and aching if he reads too long evenings by light. Aching in the upper border of the orbits, with tearing pain in the balls.

As if sight had been strained by too much reading. Dimness before the eyes like a floating shadow.

Clinical. One of the most frequently indicated remedies in asthenopia. Any of the asthenopic symptoms, as heat, and aching in and over the eyes, eyes feel like balls of fire at night, blurring of the vision, letters seem to run together, lachrymation, etc., which are caused or always made worse by straining the eyes at fine work or too much reading, are often relieved by a few doses of Ruta.

We must, of course, remember that a great majority of these cases are dependent upon anomalies in the refraction or accommodation, which renders the proper selection of glasses absolutely necessary before we can ameliorate the asthenopic symptoms.

Choroiditis in a myopic eye, caused from straining the eyes, has been cured. There was much pain in the eyes on trying to look at objects, heat in the eye (though it seems cold) and twitching in the ball of the eye.

Patients troubled with amblyopia from over-exertion of the eyes or even when no cause has been observed, have recovered their vision under the use of this drug.

SANGUINARIA.

Clinical. Benefit has been derived from its employment in blepharoadenitis, with a feeling of dryness under the upper lid and accumulation of mucus in the eye in the morning; also in blepharitis and catarrhal conditions of the conjunctiva, with burning in the edges of the lids, worse in the afternoon if dependent upon stricture of the lachrymal duct.

Ulcers of the cornea have also been favorably treated by this drug, used externally and internally at the same time.

SECALE CORNUTUM.

Clinical. According to Dr. Bacon, Secale was used with good results in a case of suppuration of the cornea which was aggravated by warm applications.

In the old school it has been used in five to ten grain doses for asthenopia marked by the usual symptoms:—WILLEBRAND.

The following case is reported by Käsemann:—A boy, æt. 19, was attacked with "amaurosis" (?) a few days previous to his appearance for treatment, caused from a cold. With the left eye he could see nothing, and with the right only objects held near. His sight was best from 12 noon to 6 P.M., and better in a darkened room on account of the great photophobia. There were sticking pains in and above both eyes, but no redness and only slight lachrymation. The pupil was dilated, nearly regular and sluggish. Blue and fiery points sometimes appeared before the eyes, and occasionally had spasmodic movements of the eyes. Bell. improved the pains and photophobia, but Secale[3] cured the case.

SENEGA.

Ciliæ hang full of hard mucus mornings. Evenings on walking toward the setting sun, another small sun seemed to float beneath it, on turning eyes outward it changed into a compressed oval, disappeared on bending head back and closing eyes.

Clinical. The action of Senega upon the lids is very marked in the provings, this together with its marked action upon general mucous surfaces renders its use in catarrhal ophthalmia quite obvious, as also in blepharitis, in which there is smarting and dry crusts on the lids, especially in the morning.

Beyne has found it useful in a bad case of conjunctivitis.

Gallavardin reports two cases of hypopion occurring in scrofulous subjects, in which its use was attended by favorable results.

Senega is of great importance in promoting the *absorption of lens fragments* after cataract operations or any other cause.

In addition to and corresponding with the general muscular laxity, we find remarkable symptoms of paralysis of the muscles of the eye; and it has proved most brilliantly curative in paresis of the left oculo-motor nerve, with paralysis of the superior rectus muscle, in which the patient could only see clearly by bending the head backwards, as this position relieved the confusion of double vision, which caused him to take missteps. The upper lid was very weak, falling half over the eye; difficult convergence; weak back; deficient muscular power; subject to bilious headaches. Senega^{200}, a dose every 24 hours, was given. Double vision better in a few days. Cured in a few weeks.

SEPIA.

Objective. Swelling and some redness of the right upper lid mornings. Inflammation of lids, with styes. Inflammation of eyes, which cannot endure cold water. Agglutination mornings. Lachrymation mornings and evenings.

Subjective. Aching over the eyes if he goes into bright daylight. Lids pain on waking as if too heavy to open. Itching of internal canthus morning, after waking; after rubbing, biting and severe lachrymation, and sore sensation in external canthus, which is somewhat agglutinated. Aching in the right eye, as from a grain of sand, aggravated by rubbing and pressing eyes together. Biting in the right eye evenings, with inclination of lids to forcibly close. Sticking in the left eye. Smarting pain in both eyes. Burning of eyes mornings, with weakness afternoons.

Vision. Fiery Sparks before the eyes, with great weakness. Daylight blinds the eyes and produces headache.

Clinical. Sepia is especially adapted to ophthalmic disorders, dependent upon uterine troubles, and in prescribing this drug, great reliance should be placed upon these and other accessory symptoms.

The *aggravation morning and evening*, and the amelioration in the middle of the day, are almost always present.

In blepharitis, both acute and chronic, good results have been obtained, especially if the above aggravation is present, and the lids are raw and sore, eyes full of matter, eversion of the puncta, numb pain in the inner canthus, etc. Also in a case, in which spasmodic entropion was present, with soreness at the internal canthi and scratching in the eyes, worse at night and at any time during the day upon closing them, as the lids feel as if they were too tight and did not cover the eye.

Reisig reports the case of a boy, about 12, in whom many little tumors were found on the lower lids, the results of styes, which impeded the movements of the lids. Sep.^{30} caused them to inflame, suppurate and disappear.

In inflammatory affections of an asthenic character, conjunctiva of a dull red color, some photophobia and swelling of the lids, worse in the mornings, we frequently find Sepia very useful.

Acute catarrhal conjunctivitis, with *drawing sensation* in the external canthus and smarting in the eyes, ameliorated by bathing in cold water and *aggravated, morning and evening*, also conjunctivitis with muco-purulent discharge in the morning and great dryness in the evening, have been quickly relieved.

It is sometimes indicated in pustular conjunctivitis, though not as frequently as when the cornea is implicated, as will be spoken of later.

Occasionally cures trachoma, with or without pannus, especially in tea-drinking females. There is often excessive irritability of the eye to both use and light, particularly worse night and morning, better through the day; lids close in spite of him and sparks may be flashing before the eyes.

For keratitis phlyctenularis, especially in females suffering from uterine disturbances, Sepia is of great value. The pains are usually of a drawing, aching or sticking character, aggravated by rubbing, pressing the lids together or pressing upon the eye. The light of day dazzles and causes the head to ache, with lachrymation, especially in the open air. The conjunctiva may be swollen, with considerable purulent discharge, edges of lids raw and sore, eruption on the face, etc. The usual time of aggravation is present.

Dr. Liebold has used it with very favorable results in keratitis parenchymatosa, complicated with uterine troubles.

A case of astigmatism resulting from granular lids, in which on reading, black seemed gray and in which the sight was better on looking out under the brows, and pain was present on using the eyes by artificial light, terminated in recovery under the use of Sepia.

At Dr. Woodyatt's suggestion, we have employed Sepia in several cases of cataract, especially in women, with manifest advantage, arresting the progress of the disease and often improving the vision very decidedly. According to H. Goullon, Jr., the following symptoms found in a lady, æt. 67, suffering from incipient hard cataract were relieved by Sep.[3]:—Was suddenly attacked, after taking cold, with pressing pain around the eyes, which is worse in the open air; before the eyes she sees constantly dark figures, like spider web lace, of the size of a hand; she has been subject to sick-headaches all her life.

Gerson reports two cases occurring in women, after change

of life, in which the following symptoms were present. The palpebral conjunctiva was injected on awaking in the morning and there was a purulent-like secretion from the glands of the lids, which continued during the forenoon, at which time there was neither pain nor photophobia. Towards evening the eyes always became dry, with biting, gnawing pains in the lids and photophobia. Later the pains were of a burning character and the lids would close tightly with entire suppression of the tears; pulse hard and rapid, and dull pain in the forehead. Would be very agitated and cry out during the paroxysm. After midnight the secretion would commence when the pains would cease. Sediment in the urine and other accessory symptoms. Sepia produced prompt relief.

Obscuration of vision dependent upon hepatic derangement, may often call for this drug.

SILICEA.

Objective. Redness of the whites of the eyes with pressive pain. An ulcer on the left eye. Agglutination nights with smarting in the lids. Lachrymation and a kind of ulceration of the eyes. Swelling in region of lachrymal gland and of lachrymal sac.

Subjective. Aching in the upper lid with severe stitches in it, as from a splinter, with vanishing of sight.

Clinical. Blepharitis with agglutination mornings, objects seem as if in a fog, relieved by wiping the eyes (Euphras.); fluent coryza, corners of the mouth cracked, with psoriasis on the arm has been cured, and shows in what form of inflammation of the lids Sil. is useful.

Boils around the eye and the lids, frequently call for this remedy; and it has also been given with advantage in cystic tumors of the lids, as reported by Stens, Sr., in A. H. Z. (Compare Staph.)

In diseases of the lachrymal apparatus it is a remedy of prime importance. It is especially adapted to inflammation of the lachrymal sac (dacryocystitis), characterized by all the prominent symptoms, swelling, tenderness, pain, lachrymation, etc., and several cases, even though well advanced so that suppuration seemed inevitable, have been cured without breaking externally, and without the aid of an operation. But, notwithstanding, experience shows how much may be sometimes gained from the administration of Silicea and other remedies, yet we would not advise delay in opening the canaliculus as soon as pus has begun to form.

Blennorrhœa of the lachrymal sac has quite frequently been controlled, and Sil. should be one of the first remedies thought of in connection with this trouble.

The treatment of acute lachrymal fistulæ by Sil. has been attended with favorable results, but chronic cases do not seem to yield to this or any other drug.

It has been recommended in traumatic ophthalmia.

Is especially indicated in sloughing ulcers of the cornea, either with or without hypopion, in small round ulcers, which have a tendency to perforate and also in non-vascular ulcers centrally located. The pains, photophobia and lachrymation, are not particularly marked. The discharge is frequently very profuse, though it may be moderate in quantity. But there is almost always present in these cases (in fact in the majority of ophthalmic disorders which call for Silicea) a great sensitiveness to cold and desire to be warmly wrapped, especially about the head.

Silicea has removed opacity of the cornea, resulting from keratitis, after small pox (!) (H. M. 6. 67.)

Schlosser reports a case of parenchymatous iritis with abscess in the upper part of the iris, violent supra-orbital pain, night and day, etc., cured by Sil.[3]

For hypopion it is especially valuable.

Many cases of so-called cataract are to be found in our journals, in which brilliant cures have been effected under Sil., though we entertain grave doubts regarding the correctness of the diagnosis. We may, however, check the progress of cataract in some cases with this remedy, when indicated by concomitant symptoms, upon which we are compelled to rely in prescribing for this affection.

The following case of sclero-choroiditis ant. was effectually relieved by this remedy. The conjunctiva and sclera were both injected and a bluish irregular bulging around the cornea was present. The retina was hazy, though no vitreous opacities were visible. There were severe pains extending from the eyes into the head, relieved by warmth, also a severe aching in the back of the head on one side, corresponding to that eye which is worse, for the severity of the symptoms alternate from one eye to the other.

It has also proved useful in choroiditis in a myope, in whom upon any exertion of the eye excessive pain extended to the head and ears.

Dr. Woodyatt recommends and has used with advantage Sil. in irido-choroiditis and other forms of inflammation of the uveal tract.

Ciliary neuralgia, characterized by darting pains through the eyes and head upon exposure to any draught of air or just before a storm, has been relieved.

In amblyopia resulting from the suppression of an habitual foot sweat, vision was restored.—BECKER.

SPIGELIA.

Objective. Lids lax and paralyzed, they hang low down and must be raised with the hand, with dilated pupils. Mornings redness and inflammation in the white of the eye; the lids seem so heavy that he can scarcely open them. Redness of the white of the eye. Lachrymation.

Subjective. Pain as if the upper lid were hard or immovable, he cannot raise it easily. Fine painful cutting on the margin of the left lower lid, like a knife. Sticking pressure under both lids. Pain as if the left orbit would be pressed together from above downward. *Constant sticking pain in the right ball. Severe boring stitch in the middle of the eye* and in the inner canthus, with drooping of the upper lid. Pain in the eye and over it. Cannot turn the left eye in all directions without pain. Eyes ache on motion as if too large for the orbits. Burning pain in the left eye toward the temples. Unendurable pressive pain in the balls, worse on turning the eyes; dizziness on turning eyes to look; he must turn the whole body to look sideways. Burning pain in the eyes, must involuntarily close them, with inner anxiety as though she would never open them again; after this pain left, the vision prevented by a sea of fire in blood red masses before the eyes; then with lachrymation and dilatation of the pupil, sight returned.

Vision. Weakness and dimness of vision; sparks before the eyes.

Clinical. This drug is especially applicable to severe neuralgic pains, arising in a great variety of ophthalmic troubles, but particularly in rheumatic and arthritic inflammations. In all cases the character and intensity of the pains furnish the chief indications for the selection of this remedy.

Ptosis, as we should be led to suppose from the symptomatology, should often require the use of Spigelia, and a case occurring in a seamstress after inflammation, with sharp stabbing pains through the eyes and head, and much hot scalding lachrymation, was very favorably affected by its use.

Is rarely called for in simple catarrhal ophthalmia, though in one case in which the left eye was affected, with lachrymation, photophobia, injection of the conjunctiva, severe sticking pain in the eye and left temple, worse at night so cannot sleep, Spig.^{200} cured.—LIPPE.

Occasionally of benefit in scrofulous conjunctivitis and keratitis, if accompanied by sharp pains, etc.

Pulte relates the following case:—A man had a pterygium develop from the inner canthus, and extend in the right eye some distance on the cornea, two years ago after a severe pain. At the present time complained of pain in the left eye as though it would fly into pieces, aggravated on stooping and always worse in the morning, continuing till noon, then suddenly disappearing. Nux vom. failed, but Spig.^{30} cured.

From the nature of the pains we not rarely employ this medicine in iritis and with excellent results, especially in the rheumatic form, with pains around and deep in the eye.

The pains of glaucoma are frequently relieved, and benefit has also been derived from its use in sclero-choroiditis, if accompanied by much pain.

Has been beneficial in strabismus with decided worm symptoms, even when some amblyopia has been present.—HIRSCH. Gallavardin also recommends its use in strabismus dependent upon worms, with neuralgic convulsions, paralytic symptoms, eclampsia, affections of the right heart, palpitation of the heart, and predominant venous and nervous erethismus.

In accommodative asthenopia, with slight retinitis and severe neuralgic headaches; also in asthenopia, with anæmia of the optic nerve and characteristic pains dependent upon too great indulgence in tea, great benefit has been obtained from Spig.

It is, however, in ciliary neuralgia, intermittent or not intermittent, dependent upon some observable disease or arising from some cause unknown, that the greatest power of Spig. is exercised. The pains are various in character, though usually *sharp and stabbing like a knife, sticking through the ball back into the head, or they may seem to start from one point and then radiate in different directions, are generally aggravated by motion and at night.* The following variety of pains, in addition to those already given, as described by patients, have been cured by Spigelia:—Pains around and deep in the eye. Severe pain on moving the eyes, worse at night. Severe pressure extending to the orbit after sleep, or as if the eye would ulcerate. Very severe sharp pain in and around the left eye, seems as if it would drive him crazy, wakes him at 3 A.M., and continues the remainder of the night; also has a similar attack in the latter part of the forenoon, always accompanied by fever and sweat. Sharp pain through the right eye and corresponding side of head, worse at night and relieved by warmth, accompanied by excessive sensitiveness of the eyeball to touch. Burning or sticking pains in the eye, and sensation as if the eyeball were too large. Burning pains going to the bones.

Sticking, boring pains extend to the bones around the eyes, especially supra-orbital and temporal regions. Eye feels too large and as if forcibly turned around in the orbit; the pain makes one shut the eye, and on opening it, seems to see a sea ot fire; with the severe pain, hot tears run out of the eye, and the pains are worse in the open air and at night. After long continued use of the eyes, terrible pains every morning at six in the left eye, as if the ball was too large and was forcibly pressed out of the orbit, with violent aching, boring and severe stitches made worse by opening and moving the eye, often extending to the forehead. The slightest touch excites the pains, which disappear about noon. Severe boring pain deep in the eye, aggravated on moving it, parts around the eye painful to touch, and sparks before the vision. Sharp sticking pains through the ball of the eye into the head on the right side, and worse at night, frontal headache and frequent winking. Intolerable pain in the supra-ciliary ridge, worse on any change of weather and in the wind. Severe pressing, jerking, sticking pains in the left eye, so hard as to cause her to cry out and lose consciousness; every few minutes would extend to the muscles of the left upper arm.

SPONGIA.

Lids torn wide open, eyes protrude, staring. Lachrymation. Heaviness of the lids. Tension around the left eye near the temple. Burning in the left eye around the ball.

On closing the lids sees sights. Objects appear in flames at night.

Clinical. Kirsten recommends Spongia very highly in maculæ of the cornea.

Its chief power has, however, been shown in Basedow's disease, as the following case will illustrate:—A woman, about forty. Eyeballs staring and perceptibly protruding; stitches in the balls and burning around the eyes, with lachrymation, worse from any sudden light; often the eye feels as if twisted around; there is constant flashing of different colors, mostly deep red, figures of light, etc., even when the eye is closed, especially at night. The thyroid gland is considerably hypertrophied. The palpitation of the heart is very marked, which makes her uneasy, restless and easily frightened, especially at night. Spongia in the higher potencies effected a cure.

Hirsch reports a well marked case of exophthalmus, which Spong.[2] relieved.

STANNUM.

Pustular swelling in the inner canthus of the left eye, like a lachrymal fistula.

Pressive pain in the inner canthus. Biting in the eyes, as from rubbing with a woolen cloth.

Clinical. Stannum has been employed by Drs. Liebold and Hunt in blennorrhœa of the lachrymal sac, with advantage in controlling the amount of the discharge.

STAPHYSAGRIA.

Pimples around the inflamed eye. Biting, smarting pain in the internal canthus. Dryness evenings, and aching. Eyes ache soon on writing (afternoons); biting and burning, then biting lachrymation and photophobia.

Clinical. Especially applicable to affections of the lids, being very rarely used in other diseases of the eye.

The form of blepharitis to which Staphysagria is adapted may be found, when the margins of the lids are dry with hard lumps on their borders and destruction of the hair follicles.

Its greatest usefulness is in tarsal tumors in which it is quite commonly employed, as when the glands of the lids are enlarged with redness, and tensive tearing pains, especially in the evening, or more particularly if little hard nodules are found on the lids, resulting from styes, also if crops of small tarsal tumors are constantly recurring.

Anchylops, appearing every month just before the full moon, leaving behind a small hard tumor and accompanied by tensive, tearing pains extending from the eye to the teeth and cheek of corresponding side, worse at night with headache, sneezing, coryza, etc., was permanently cured by Staph.[15].—HAUBOLD.

Syphilitic iritis with bursting pain in the eyeball, temple and side of face, worse from evening to morning and upon using the eyes by any light, was promptly relieved by this drug.—BACON.

Six cases of "arthritic ophthalmia" are on record as cured, in which the pains extended from the eyes to the teeth on one side, with burning in the eyes on the slightest exertion as though they were very dry, although constant lachrymation was present.

STRAMONIUM.

Greatest sensitiveness to daylight and desire for lamplight.

Objects appear oblique.—

Clinical. Has relieved diplopia, and Gallavardin recommends its use in strabismus from brain affections, epilepsy, eclampsia or chorea, if aggravated by mental exertion, terror or fear.

SULPHUR.

Objective. Painful pimples over the brows. Intense red, severely itching and burning spot on skin of left external canthus. Copious discharge from meibomian glands. Lids red and caruncles much congested. Stye on the upper lid at the inner canthus. Swelling of the upper lid, with dry matter in the lashes. Redness of the lids and conjunctiva. Conjunctiva and sclera much congested. Swelling and redness of the eyes, with eruption on the lids. White vesicle on the white of the eye, near the cornea. Lachrymation and agglutination of the eyes.

Subjective. Much itching in the brows, and tips of the

nose. Burning in the canthi and feeling of sand. By candle-light itching near the internal canthus, with stinging pain. Itching stinging in the right external canthus, with sensation as of fine sparks glimmering in the right upper lid. Itching of the lids as if they would be inflamed. Itching and burning in the lids, which are red and swollen. Sense of many burning sparks in the lids, which are immediately drawn together. Prickling, itching and biting in the lids, must scratch and rub on waking mornings. Feeling of fine sand between the right upper lid and ball. Aching in the eyes every evening as from sleepiness, without sleepiness. Balls pain on moving them. Biting in the eyes as from the fumes of sal-ammoniac. *Sticking in the eyes* (right), *as with knives. Severe pains* in the left eye, *as if it turned against a glass splinter* and forced it towards the pupil, followed by burning and lachrymation, must close the eyes.

Vision. Dimness as from a veil. Small black points. Diplopia.

Clinical. Blepharitis, particularly the chronic form, quite frequently calls for this drug, especially if occurring in children of a strumous diathesis, who are irritable and cross by day and restless and feverish by night. The lids are swollen, red and agglutinated in the morning, from the increased secretion of the meibomian glands, or there may be numerous small itching pustules on the margins. There may be itching, biting, burning or sensation as if sand were in the eye, though the pains are usually of a sticking character. There is generally great aversion to water, so cannot bear to have the eyes washed. Is especially of use when appearing after the suppression of an eruption, or if the child or adult is already covered with eczema.

Eczematous affections of the lids have been often controlled, when Sulph. has been given according to the indications for eczema in other portions of the body.

It has prevented the recurrence of successive crops of styes.

It may be found of service in blennorrhœa of the lachrymal sac, though is not frequently indicated.

Fresh lachrymal fistula with all the usual symptoms, is on record as cured.

In conjunctivitis catarrhalis, both acute and chronic, this remedy is often very useful. The degree of redness may vary greatly, be confined to one eye or involve both. The lids may be swollen, even puffy, or remain unaffected. But the sharp darting pains, like *pins sticking into the eye*, will furnish our chief indications, (these pains are characteristic of the drug and may occur at any time of the day or night). There may also be pressing, tensive, *cutting* or burning pains, feeling of sand in them, tearing in the head, poor appetite, feverishness at night, chills during the day, etc.

Trachoma, acute and chronic, has been benefited. It is often called for as an intercurrent remedy, even if it does not complete the cure alone, especially if the pains are *sharp and sticking* in the morning and the lids are glued together, so that it is with the greatest difficulty they can be opened. Water is not a favorite application and usually aggravates the trouble.

Pterygium with no especial symptoms, but supposed to be dependent upon hereditary psora, has been cured with Sulph.[3]. —B. CORNELL.

Has been employed with success in ophthalmia neonatorum, marked by the usual symptoms of profuse thick yellow discharge, swelling of the lids, etc. Is especially indicated in chronic cases that have a great tendency to relapse and when syphilis has not been the cause.

It is, however, the remedy "par excellence" for pustular inflammation of the cornea or conjunctiva, and is more frequently indicated than any other drug. Its sphere of action is very wide; it is therefore adapted to a great variety of cases, especially if chronic, and occurring in scrofulous children covered with eruptions (among which the majority of these cases are found), or when otorrhœa and diseases of the bones complicate the difficulty; also to those cases caused by suppressing an eruption with external applications. The character of the pains may vary, though they are usually *sharp and sticking, as if a needle or splinter was sticking into the eye*, or we may have a *sharp, shooting pain going through the eye back into the head, from* 1 *to* 3 *A.M.*, awakening him from sleep, although besides these we have a variety of other sensations, such as smarting, itching and burning in the eyes, a feeling of pressure as from a foreign body, burning as from lime, biting as if salt were in the eye, sensation as if there were a number of little burning sparks on the lids, which cause them to spasmodically close, painful dryness as if the lids rubbed the eyeball, bruised pain, etc., etc. The photophobia is generally very marked and the lachrymation profuse, though in some cases it may be almost or entirely absent. The redness varies greatly, but is usually considerable, especially at the angles. The secretions also vary both in quantity and quality, being often, however, acrid, corrosive, and sometimes tenacious. Agglutination in the morning is commonly present. The lids are often swollen, burn and smart, as if bathed in some acrid fluid, or there is an itching sensation, compelling the patient to rub them most of the time, they, as well as the surrounding integument of the head and face, are frequently covered with an eruption. All the symptoms are, as a rule, *aggravated by bathing the eyes* so that the child cannot bear to have any water touch them, and are worse in the open air.

The value of Sulphur in the treatment of ulcers and abscesses of the cornea, is hardly less than in pustular inflammation; its usefulness is not confined to any one species of ulcer, as it has cured not only the superficial variety, but also the deep sloughing form, which tend towards perforation and destruction of the whole cornea. In fact it should always be thought of in ulceration or abscess of the cornea, with hypopion, especially if of an indolent form, with no photophobia nor vascularity, etc., as it has often produced absorption of the pus, and exercised a beneficial influence over the destructive process going on in the cornea. The indications which lead us to its selection in this affection, are derived chiefly from the general condition of the patient, while the characteristic eye symptoms are the same as those given above for the phlyctenular form of inflammation, except in the severer forms in which the pains may be more intense, as severe pressive pains in the whole circumference of the orbit, which are worse on any movement of the eye, exposure to sunlight or any motion of the lids, even closing them causes almost unbearable pains, which extend to the whole head and deprive one of all rest and reason.—GROSS. There may be severe pressing pains in the eye besides the characteristic stitches. The other symptoms may also be proportionately increased.

Superficial keratitis with slight ulceration of the surface of the cornea, often requires the use of this remedy, and it has also been recommended for superficial ophthalmia dependent upon traumatic causes.

Pannus resulting from various causes and occurring in patients of a strumous diathesis, has been frequently cured. In some instances there has been true pannus crassum, the whole of the cornea presenting the appearance of a piece of fresh raw beef, and yet vision has been restored by the internal administration of Sulph. In one case in which the drug in a high potency cured, the patient complained that upon looking at a candle-light, there was a green halo around it.—W. D. HALL. Is especially useful in the so-called herpetic pannus, resulting from phlyctenules, etc.

A case of keratitis parenchymatosa in a scrofulous subject, cornea like ground glass, photophobia, lids swollen and bleed easily, was permanently relieved by this remedy, and it will often be found to promote absorption of the infiltration, after the disease has been checked by other remedies.

Benefit has been derived from its use in opacities of the cornea.

In severe forms of inflammation of the cornea, the iris not unfrequently becomes involved (kerato-iritis) though this does not by any means contra-indicate the use of Sulph., even if hypopion be present.

Has been employed with favorable results in inflammation of the sclera, with corneal and iritic complications, as well as in uncomplicated cases. There may be in addition to the well-known objective symptoms, only a feeling of fullness and largeness of the eyeball, worse from use or exposure to light, especially gas-light, or there may be great photophobia, acrid lachrymation and severe tearing pains in the supra-orbital and temporal regions, as well as in the eye itself, especially worse in the evening and at night.

In iritis, both idiopathic and syphilitic, (especially the former) benefit has, occasionally, been derived from the use of this remedy, though it is not frequently indicated. Is especially adapted to chronic cases marked by some drawing pain around the eye, but chiefly by *sharp sticking pains* in the eyes, worse at night (Spig.) and towards morning. The eyeball may be painful on motion, and the usual characteristic symptoms are present.

After iritis, the recent adhesions (posterior synechiæ) often give way very promptly.

The hypopion resulting from iritis, or in fact pus found in the anterior chamber under any circumstances will frequently disappear after the administration of a few doses of Sulphur.

Cataract, especially when occurring after the suppression of an eruption, has been reported cured by Kirsch, Schönfeld, Malan and others.

Hyperæmia of the retina, when general symptoms call for its use, has been benefited.

Retinitis caused from over study, with much congestion of the optic nerve, outlines ill-defined, and accompanied by pain around the eye and itching in the internal canthi, has been cured.

Its usefulness in inflammatory affections of the fundus is not confined to retinitis, as it has also been successfully employed in chorio-retinitis and uncomplicated choroiditis, if accompanied by darting pains, and in one case in which hemeralopia was present. It is not, however, a frequently indicated remedy for any of the acute forms of intra-ocular diseases (though is sometimes useful, especially as an inter-current), but is particularly called for in chronic cases. Payr says, regarding its use in choroiditis, that it is frequently indicated in the chronic form, especially when the trouble is based upon abdominal venosity, stagnation in the portal circulation, habitual constipation and cerebral congestion conditioned thereby; also in metastases of chronic or suppressed skin diseases.

Sulphur often acts very promptly in clearing up opacities in the vitreous, resulting from choroideal exudations, old hemorrhages, etc.

The following case of sympathetic irritation of the right eye occurring in a young lady, was speedily relieved:—The left eye had been removed, on account of extensive staphylomatous bulging of the whole eye, six months previous, by abscising the cornea and evacuating the contents of the globe, thus leaving only the sclera and muscles intact. She now appeared complaining of sharp pain in the stump, extending in stitches to the healthy eye, in which there was considerable irritation and photophobia, occasional obscuration of vision and commencing presbyopia. There is constant discharge from the old stump, which is excessively sensitive to touch. Sulph.^{200} relieved in a few days.

Many cases are on record, diagnosticated "ophthalmia arthritica" in which the administration of Sulph. has been followed by favorable results. In some the deep structures were involved, while in others only the superficial, though the indications leading to its choice did not vary from those already given.

Asthenopia, both muscular and accommodative, have been occasionally benefited, when the character of the pains, etc., have pointed to its selection. "Gaslight hurts more than sunlight," a symptom not rarely found in these cases, has been relieved.

Amaurosis and amblyopia, accompanied or not by diplopia, arising from the suppression of an eruption or from various causes, have been helped.

The following case of "amaurosis" occurring in a woman, æt. 48, is reported by Bethmann:—After severe tearing in the head, especially on the left side, noticed an appearance of threads before the eyes, which she could not wipe away; this increased until she could only distinguish day from night; burning, tearing in the eyes and conjunctiva slightly red. Sulphur tincture restored the vision.

The iodide of sulphur has been occasionally employed in ophthalmic diseases with marked success, especially when found in strumous subjects with enlarged glands, etc.

TABACUM.

Clinical. Gallavardin recommends its use in strabismus, dependent upon brain troubles.

Benefit has been found from its employment in asthenopia.

The following case consequent upon the use of tobacco may prove interesting:—The patient is amblyopic, vision $\frac{20}{100}$, refraction normal, divergence of $1\frac{1}{2}$ lines behind a screen, diplopia in the distance. On leaving off tobacco for a time he improves and sees single, but within ten minutes after returning to its use the vision becomes dim, black spots float before the eyes and he sees double. Stimulants only aggravate the difficulty.

TELLURIUM.

Clinical. Has proved successful in conjunctivitis pustulosa, with eczema impetiginoides on the lids and much purulent discharge from the eyes, also an offensive discharge from the ear, to which the child is subject.

It is probably more often indicated in scrofulous ophthalmia, than we are now led to suppose.

The offensive otorrhœa, smelling like fish brine is an important concomitant symptom.

TEREBINTH.

Clinical. This remedy has been successfully employed by Dr. Liebold in many cases of iritis, especially the rheumatic variety, when urinary symptoms are present, as frequent desire, pressure and pain in the kidneys, burning in the urethra, hæmaturia, etc.; also when there can be found a suppression of habitual transpiration of the feet.

Recent adhesions of the iris to the lens (posterior synechiæ) have also seemed to yield under its use.

THUYA.

Objective. Stye on the right eye, followed by inflammation. With inflammation of lids, there is dryness and itching. White scales on the lids. Ciliæ bent with small, dry, brownish scurfs. Margin of lower lid covered with red pimples. Severe redness of the conjunctiva of the ball and lids, with some swelling, lachrymation and itching, beginning evenings. Lachrymation (not running over). Pupils contracted.

Subjective. Aching over the right eye. Heat and dryness in the left external canthus, as if it would inflame. Feeling as if sand were in the eyes. Constant aching in the eye, worse in the bright light. Eyes ameliorated by warm covering, as soon as uncovered, pains and sensation as of a stream of cold from the head through them.

Photophobia. Colored flashes before the vision.

Clinical. Is useful in that form of tinea ciliaris which corresponds to pityriasis capitis, dry, bran-like eruption on the eyelids, chiefly about the ciliæ, eyelashes irregular and imperfectly grown, scales covering the skin, very fine, and the eyes weak and watery. Such are the symptoms of a case which had existed for years and was cured by Thuya.—R. F. Cooper.

Tülf says that it has cured obstinate forms of styes, when other remedies have failed.

As a remedy for tarsal tumors it is very valuable, especially for verucæ and tumors that resemble small condylomata, though it may be useful for other forms, not only, as recommended by some, in preventing their return after removal by the knife, but also, in promoting their absorption without the employment of instrumental means. This can not unfrequently be done by simply using the drug internally, though in some cases it has seemed to act quicker if employed in the tincture externally at the same time.

Fungoid growths are also said to have been helped.—Hartung.

Old chronic catarrhal conjunctivitis, always worse after being disturbed of his usual rest at night, has been relieved.—A. K. Frain.

Conjunctivitis trachomatosa, in which the granulations are large like warts or blisters, with burning in the lids and eyes, worse at night, photophobia by day and suffusion of the eye in tears, would lead us to give Thuya with favorable results.

Has been occasionally found of use in inflammations of the cornea, especially in ulcerations of a syphilitic origin, even if hypopion is present.

The following interesting case is reported by Kunkel in A. H. Z.:—A girl about eleven, scrofulous diathesis, lost her sight seven years ago. There is now total leucomatous dimness of both corneæ, conjunctiva injected and lids spasmodically closed, especially in the daylight; the photophobia is intense so cannot open the lids, the light even hurts the eye when closed, worse at 5 P.M.; sticking and tearing in the eyes evenings, constant flow of salty water, lids appear normal; is very restless and sleepless until along towards morning, when she obtains a little rest; often after 4 P.M. she has fever, chills, thirst and sweat; appetite fair, though pain in the stomach after eating; frequent vertigo without congestion; always has cold feet. Thuya^{30} caused a purulent discharge, which cured the case, with the exception of a slight opacity of the cornea.

An interesting case of vascular tumor of the cornea, which covered nearly two-thirds of its inner surface, is reported by Dr. Drysdale as cured with Thuya^{30} internally, and the first externally.

The action of Thuya upon the sclera is very marked indeed, probably more so than any other drug, and it has been employed with excellent success in *episcleritis*, sclero-choroiditis ant. and commencing scleral staphyloma, even when no characteristic indications were present.

For syphilitic iritis, marked by *condylomata on the iris*, it is a grand remedy. The pains are usually severe, sharp and sticking in the eye, worse at night, with *much heat* above and around the eye, or there may be a pain in the left frontal eminence, as if a nail were being driven in; in some cases the pain is expressed as a dull aching in the eye, and sometimes seems to be relieved in the open air. There may also be present suffusion of the eyes in tears, burning in the lids and eyes, stitching pain in the temples, noises in the head, etc.

Exophthalmus consequent upon a tumor behind the eyeball has been relieved.

In a case of amblyopia with blurring of the vision relieved by rubbing (Euphras.), black spots and bright sparks before the eyes, and dull aching above the eye to the back of the head, with nausea, the vision was restored by this remedy.

The following symptoms of vision have also been relieved:— "Flames of light before the eyes mostly yellow," and "when looking into the light of day, sees white spots like bottles of water moving about."

VERATRUM ALBUM.

Clinical. Cured a case of hemeralopia with nightly diarrhœa, in a boy, ten years of age.

VIOLA ODORATA.

Clinical. Stapf reports the following symptoms found in a woman, æt. 26, as relieved by Viola od.^{200}:—Toward evening a feeling of dryness and burning in the lids; sensitiveness to light; painful forcible drawing together of the lids as from irresistible sleep. No disease to be discovered in the lids.

VIOLA TRICOLOR.

Clinical. Dudgeon has found it of service in scrofulous ophthalmia with crusta lactea. Lids much swollen, and soft parts around so much inflamed that the lids cannot be opened. Face covered with a raw looking, excoriating eruption.

ZINCUM.

Objective. Inflammation and redness of the conjunctiva of the right eye, and matter in the inner canthus. The eye pains most evening and night, as from sand in it; frequent lachrymation; the upper lid is too red and swollen toward the inner canthus. Lachrymation in conjunctivitis.

Subjective. Sudden painful pressure over the right eye, with pressing down feeling in the lids. Painful aching in the right inner canthus and redness of the conjunctiva. Biting in the inner canthus of right eye, ameliorated by rubbing. Sore feeling in the inner canthus. Burning and biting, with photophobia and lachrymation evenings, and agglutination mornings. Unendurable pain in the left eye, great restlessness and frequent great weakness in the head.

Clinical. Has been especially employed in diseases of the conjunctiva.

For pterygium in particular, it is a valuable remedy, as several well marked cases have been cured. In one case reported by Dr. Dunham, the pterygium covered one half of the pupil and was growing rapidly; there was much conjunctival injection, lachrymation in the evening, discharge and photophobia, especially by artificial light, pricking pain and soreness, worse in the inner angle and in the evening, but particularly marked was a sensation of *great pressure across the root of the nose* and supra-orbital region. Zincum cured. In another case of pterygium, which nearly covered the cornea, there was photophobia and profuse lachrymation at night, external canthi cracked, much itching and heat in the eye at night, worse in the cold air and better in a warm room; she sees a green halo around the evening light, and has attacks of rush of blood to the head, etc. Under Zinc.^{200}, the green halo first disappeared, then the lachrymation, aggravation nights, etc.

Has been useful in conjunctivitis, especially if confined to the inner half of the eye, usually without photophobia. Has also removed persistent redness of the conjunctiva, remaining after pustular keratitis, without any discharge, worse towards evening and in the cool air.

Kerato-iritis with severe night pains, especially in the inner angle of the eye, has been benefited.

Syphilitic iritis with dull pain in the balls and brows, coming on as soon as he lies down at night, and accompanied by profuse, hot scalding lachrymation, was speedily cured by Zinc.^{200}.

Periodic and temporary amaurosis or amblyopia, occurring during severe attacks of headache, and passing away with the headache, are on record as cured. Kafka reports one case which had continued two years, occurring every two weeks, and lasting from two to three days. The attacks came on suddenly, with severe pressure in the vertex, and forehead, from without inwards, and were worse in the afternoon and evening. The amblyopia appeared as a thick cloud, grew worse until she became completely blind, and then disappeared with the pain. Face pale, appetite poor, very irritable, Zinc., 3d dil., cured.

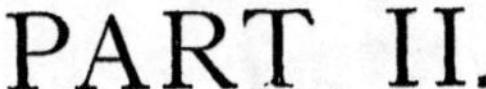

PART II.

OPHTHALMIC

THERAPEUTICS.

ORBIT.

PERIOSTITIS, CARIES AND NECROSIS OF THE ORBIT.

The line of treatment laid down for cellulitis, applies very well to the above, as we should at first endeavor to prevent destruction of tissue, but if that does occur, give the pus free vent; also the remedies described under cellulitis, are applicable to this disease; in addition, we note the following:—

Aurum for both periostitis and *caries*, when *dependent upon or complicated with a mercurio-syphilitic dyscrasia;* also useful in strumous subjects. The pains are tense, and seem to be in the bones, are worse at night, bone sensitive to touch, and the patient is excessively sensitive to the pain.

Calc. hypophos. in appreciable doses, has been used as a "tissue remedy" in scrofulous subjects, apparently with good results.

Kali iod. This form of potash is a frequent remedy in old mercurial cases, and where syphilis is the cause of the difficulty.

Mercurius. As described under cellulitis, this remedy will be found very useful in both periostitis and caries, particularly when dependent upon syphilis, as the nocturnal aggravation is very marked under both the drug and disease. The different forms are employed according to general indications.

The following remedies have also been found very useful:—Asaf., Carb. an., Caust., Fluoric ac., *Hecla lava.*, Lyc., Mang. ac., Mez., Nat. mur., Nit. ac., Petrol., Ruta, Rhod., Staphys., *Sil.* and Sulphur.

CELLULITIS ORBITÆ.

When this form of inflammation results from an injury or the introduction of a foreign body, the latter should be first removed, and then cold compresses of Calendula solution employed to subdue the inflammatory symptoms. But if suppuration has already set in, poultices should be applied to promote the discharge of pus, which should be evacuated *at an early period*, by a free incision through the conjunctiva if practicable, if not, through the lid itself. Care should be taken that the pus has free vent at all times. Diet and rest will be prescribed according to the general tone of the patient and severity of the attack.

Aconite in the first stage, when the lids are much swollen with a tight feeling in them, conjunctiva chemosed, and much *heat* and *sensitiveness* in and around the eye, with a sensation as if the eyeball were protruding, making the lids tense, associated with the general Aconite fever.

Apis mel. Before the formation of pus. *Lids œdematously swollen, with stinging, shooting pains.* Patient drowsy, without thirst.

Hepar sulph. Especially after pus has formed. Lids swollen and *very sensitive to both touch and cold.* Pains are severe and of a *throbbing* character.

Lachesis. Orbital cellulitis following squint operation, point of tenotomy sloughing, with a *black spot in the centre;* conjunctiva chemosed, much discharge with general Lach. condition.

Mercurius. In the later stages after pus has formed, and even after it has discharged for some time and has become *thin* in character, especially when occurring in a syphilitic subject. There is often much pain in and around the eye, always worse at night.

Rhus tox. Is a remedy of the very first importance in this form of inflammation, whether or not of traumatic origin. *The lids are œdematously swollen, as well as the conjunctiva*, and upon opening them, a profuse gush of tears takes place. The pa ns vary in character, and are usually greatly influenced by any change in the weather. See under Rhus.

Other remedies may be thought of, as Ars., Bell., Bry., Kali hyd., Sil., Sulph.

MORBUS BASEDOWII.

(*Exophthalmic Goitre.*)

We are compelled to place our chief reliance upon internal remedies in the treatment of this disorder, though there are several means which may be employed as adjuvants, as galvanization of the sympathetic in the neck, which has been employed with very good success in many instances, especially when combined with internal medication.

Both tarsoraphy and tenotomy of the levator palpebræ superioris, have been advised and employed in order to protect the partially uncovered globe.

These proceedings are, however, of very questionable utility. To promote a permanent cure, rest, especially in the country, freedom from all excitement, especially emotional, exercise in open air, a generous diet and abstinence from all stimulants, are particularly required, and should be insisted upon whenever practicable.

Amyl nit. Cases have been entirely cured by olfaction of this drug alone. The eyes are protruding, staring, and the conjunctival vessels injected, as well as those of the fundus. Especially indicated when there are frequent flushes of the face and head, oppressed respiration, etc.

Cactus grand. Prescribed from the heart symptoms, cases of exophthalmic goitre have been improved.

Chloroform. Is said to have improved a case occurring in a woman, which came on after the administration of Chloroform.

Ferrum. Both the iodide and acetate have been followed by favorable results, especially when coming on after the suppression of the menses, protruding eyes, enlargement of the thyroid, palpitation of the heart and excessive nervousness.

Lycopus virg. Should, judging from its provings, be a valuable remedy in this disorder. But, though experience gives us some good results, they are not as great as one would be led to suppose.

Spongia. Exophthalmus, enlargement of thyroid and palpitation of heart, great uneasiness and easily frightened, especially at night; stitches in the ball and burning around the eyes, with lachrymation when in the light; often the eye feels twisted around; chromopsis (especially deep red) and photopsies, even when the eye is closed at night, indicate this drug, which has proved valuable.

Nat. mur. and Baryta c., are reported to have cured well marked cases.

Other remedies which have been recommended, are Bell., Brom., Calc., Iod., Phos., Sil. and Sulph.

TUMORS OF THE ORBIT.

The most common method of treatment of all tumors of the orbit, is to remove them as early as possible, whenever practicable, endeavoring to save the eye whenever sight is present, unless it be a malignant growth and there is danger of not removing the whole of the tumor without sacrificing the globe; in which case it is usually better to remove all the contents of the orbit.

Our remedies are the same as for tumors in other portions of the body, though we would especially mention *Thuya*, which has been of service in some cases.

WOUNDS AND INJURIES OF THE ORBIT.

When a foreign body has penetrated the orbit, it should be removed as soon as possible; after which apply cold compresses of Calendula in solution.

If there has been an effusion of blood into the orbit, as the result of an injury, or when spontaneous (as is rarely the case), causing the eye to protrude, a cold compress and a firm bandage will be found very beneficial.

LACHRYMAL APPARATUS.

DISEASES OF THE LACHRYMAL GLAND.

Affections of this gland, acute and chronic inflammation, hypertrophy, fistulæ, tumors, etc., are of rare occurrence, and the treatment does not vary from analogous diseases in other portions of the body.

DACRYO-CYSTITIS.

At the commencement of an inflammation of the lachrymal sac, before the formation of pus has begun, cold compresses, (even ice) are advisable, which, together with the indicated remedy, may cause the inflammation to abort before an abscess has formed.

As soon, however, as pus has begun to collect in the lachrymal sac, our treatment must undergo a decided change. The first and most important step to be taken, is the *opening of the canaliculus* into the sac; evacuate its contents and give the pus free exit through this, its natural channel. This, as we have said, must be done as soon as suppuration is suspected, for if not attended to, an opening externally will be made, and a lachrymal fistula may be the result.

(Probing of the nasal duct should be avoided until the severity of the inflammation has subsided.) Warm applications should now be substituted for the cold. Among the best of those in use, we consider a solution of Calendula, which should be applied warm.

Internal medication during the whole course of the disease, will form an important feature in the treatment. *Acon.*, *Puls.*, *Sil.* and *Hepar*, are most commonly called for, but for special indications, refer to "blennorrhœa of the lachrymal sac."

Under this treatment the inflammatory symptoms usually

disappear, though a catarrhal condition of the lachrymal sac may remain behind, which requires further treatment.

If the patient neglects to apply for treatment until the abscess has opened spontaneously, or until perforation is iminent, it is best to make a free incision externally, treat by warm compresses, etc., and then later open the canaliculus and close the fistulous opening.

BLENNORRHŒA OF THE LACHRYMAL SAC AND STRICTURE OR CLOSURE OF THE LACHRYMAL DUCT.

Since this disease is frequently dependent upon nasal catarrh, treatment must be directed to this affection; if aggravated by the presence of nasal polypi, or caused by foreign bodies, these must, of course, be removed.

Our first indication is to prevent the collection of tears and diseased secretions in the sac. To accomplish this, it is best to slit up the canaliculus, thus giving the secretions free vent.

For stricture of the lachrymal duct. Slight or moderate strictures, (almost always dependent upon catarrhal inflammation) must be treated by appropriate medication, from which better results will be finally obtained than from probing. If the stricture is so great as to almost close the duct, it is better to proceed as in cases of complete closure. Probing for a long time, using larger and larger probes, is highly recommended by allopathic authorities, and is often followed by temporary benefit.

If the matter continues to collect in the sac, the patient must be instructed to press it out several times a day; he should also avoid anything that tends to produce irritation, such as cold winds and over-exertion of the eyes.

If there is closure of the nasal duct or a firm stricture, it should be divided. In order to prevent adhesions after the operation, we have found the use of leaden probes of great value; during the first week after the operation, the largest size should be introduced every other day and allowed to remain in twelve hours (or over night). After this they may be introduced at increasing intervals of one week, two weeks, one month, two months. In the meantime, having the catarrhal inflammation under treatment.

Aconite. Inflammation of the lachrymal sac, with great heat, dryness, tenderness, sharp pains and general fever.

Arum. triph. Catarrh of the lachrymal sac with desire to bore into the side of the nose; nose obstructed, compelled to breathe through the mouth; watery discharge from the nose, but at the same time obstructed, especially in the morning. Nostrils sore; the left discharges continually.

Argentum nit. Discharge very profuse, caruncula lachrymalis swollen, looking like a lump of red flesh; conjunctiva usually congested.

Argentum met. relieved a case of stricture.

Calendula. As a local application in blennorrhœa of the sac, after the canaliculus had been opened, has at times been found useful, especially in cases of great tenderness.

Euphrasia. Much *thick*, *yellow*, *acrid discharge*, making the lids sore and excoriated. Blurring of the vision relieved by winking; thin, watery *bland* discharge from the nose.

Hepar sulph. Inflammation of the lachrymal sac after pus had formed, or in blennorrhœa, with great sensitiveness to touch and to cold, with profuse discharge.

Mercurius. Discharge thin and excoriating, acrid coryza, nocturnal aggravation.

Petroleum. Discharge from the lachrymal sac, with roughness of the cheek, occipital headache, and other marked concomitant symptoms.

Pulsatilla. Dacryocystitis may sometimes be cut short at its very beginning, with this. Is also important in blennorrhœa of the sac, if the *discharge is profuse and bland.* Profuse thick and bland discharge from the nose.

Silicea. Very commonly indicated in dacryocystitis characterized by the usual symptoms; even cases that have far advanced toward suppuration, have been checked. Blennorrhœa of the lachrymal sac often calls for it. The patient is particularly sensitive to cold air and wishes to keep warmly covered.

Other remedies which have been recommended and proved useful are Bell., Calc., *Cinnab.*, Cimicif., Con., Hydrast., Kali iod., *Nat. mur.*, Sanguin., Stram., Stilling., and Sulph.

FISTULA LACHRYMALIS.

The first point to be attended to, is to see that the passage is free into the nose; we must therefore slit up the canaliculus and divide any stricture found in the nasal duct, providing it is sufficient to interfere with the passage of the tears into the nose; after which, this should be kept open.

The fistula must now be healed, and if recent, this is best done by touching the edges with a stick of nitrate of silver. Packing it with alumen exsiccatum has also proved of advantage. If the edges of the fistula are healed and covered with smooth skin, it will be necessary to pare the edges and unite with a suture.

The following remedies have been advised and may have been of service in recent cases, though we doubt if any effect can be obtained in old chronic cases. Brom., Calc., Fluoric ac., Lach., Nat. mur., Petrol., Sil. and Sulph.

LIDS.

ŒDEMA OF THE LIDS.

As this condition is usually dependent upon some constitutional cause or severer forms of inflammation of the conjunctiva, cornea, or iris, it should be considered as only a symptom which will disappear when the original trouble subsides. We are, however, frequently called upon for relief of this troublesome and disfiguring symptom, often when no special cause can be readily found. Our remedies are generally all we require for its removal, though a compress bandage may materially assist in some instances. The chief remedies are, *Apis*, *Ars.*, *Kali carb. and Rhus.*

(For special indications, see part 1.)

BLEPHARITIS ACUTA (ABSCESSUS PALPEBRÆ).

By a careful selection of our remedy in the first stage, we can often cause the inflammation to subside before suppuration has taken place. It is also possible to promote the resolution and discharge of pus already formed. Cold (iced) applications are recommended if the disease is seen at the outset; but if we suspect that the formation of pus has commenced, a change to hot applications (poultices) should be made.

As soon as fluctuation can be felt, a free incision into the swelling parallel to the margin of the lid, should be made, in order to give free vent to the confined pus. After the escape of the pus, warm applications of Calendula and water (ten drops to the ounce) are advised. A compress bandage should also be employed if the abscess is extensive, so as to keep the lid in position and the walls of the abscess in contact, and thus hasten the union.

If it has already spontaneously opened, the perforation should be enlarged if it be insufficient, and unfavorably situated; also if there be several apertures, they should be united by an incision, in order to leave as small a cicatrix as possible. A generous diet should be prescribed.

Aconite. In the *very first stage*, when the lids are swollen, red, hard, and with a tight feeling in them; also when they are very *sensitive to air* and touch, with *great heat* and burning. There is hardly any lachrymation present. General febrile symptoms often accompany the above.

Apis mel. Incipient stage, before the formation of pus, if there is *great puffiness of the lids, especially of the upper, with stinging pains.* Much swelling of the lids of a reddish blue color; temporary relief from cold water. The conjunctiva is often chemosed and the lachrymation profuse, hot, and burning, (Rhus), though not acrid as under Arsenicum. Drowsiness and absence of thirst are often present.

Arsenicum. When the inflammation of the lids is dependent upon, or associated with a general cachectic habit, great prostration, restlessness, especially at night, much thirst, etc. The lids may be œdematously swollen, especially the lower, though not usually very red. *The pains are of a decided burning character*, and the *lachrymation profuse, hot, and acrid*, excoriating the lids and cheek.

Hepar sulph. This is the remedy most frequently employed, especially after the first stage has passed, and *suppuration is about to, or has already taken place.*

The lids are inflamed, as if erysipelas had invaded them, with throbbing, aching, stinging pain in them, and are very sensitive to touch; the pains are aggravated by cold and from contact, but ameliorated by warmth.

The lowest preparations promote the formation of pus and its determination toward the surface. The higher potencies prevent suppuration and promote absorption.

Rhus tox. When there is a tendency to the formation of an abscess; lids œdematously swollen (especially the upper) and accompanied by *profuse lachrymation;* there may be *erysipelatous swelling* of lids with vesicles on the skin. *Conjunctiva often* *chemosed.* The pains are worse at night, and in cold, damp weather, but relieved by warm applications.

Silicea. Indicated after suppuration has commenced. Silicea is more particularly called for in the carbuncular form, and especially if the patient is very nervous and the local symptoms accompanied by sharp pains in the head ameliorated by wrapping up warm.

Graph., Iris vers., Psor., *Puls.*, Sep., Staph. and *Sulph.*, are said to have been of service. The special indications are to be found under blepharitis ciliaris.

BLEPHARITIS CILIARIS.

(Syn. tinea tarsi, ophthalmia tarsi, blepharitis marginalis, seu tarsalis, blepharoadenitis, etc. Including acne ciliaris, eczema palpebrarum and phtheiriasis ciliarum.)

"Tolle causam" should be our motto in contending against this trouble; for, unless the causes are removed, (and they are many) no headway can be made in the treatment.

First, we should, as a rule, examine the refraction of the patient, whether he be hypermetropic or myopic, for often we find this to be the chief cause (especially hypermetropia), particularly when there is only slight inflammation of the edge of the lids, giving them a red, irritable look, with little scurfs on the ciliæ. In these cases, the first thing to do is to correct the anomaly of refraction by prescribing the proper glass, which is sometimes sufficient to cure the whole trouble, though we may afterwards need some external application or internal medication in addition.

In rare cases the presence of lice on the eyelashes, may be the exciting cause, (phtheiriasis ciliarum) when we should be careful to remove them, and apply either cosmoline or some mercurial ointment, which will destroy them and prevent their recurrence.

Fungous growths in the hair follicles, are also said to cause this disease, in which case the hairs should be extirpated, and either external or internal medication employed.

Blepharitis ciliaris is often developed secondarily after some other trouble of the eye, as conjunctivitis, keratitis, etc., besides being often found as a sequela of acute exanthemata, as small-pox, measles, etc.

In some persons there seems to be a pre-disposition to this trouble, for it will occur after almost any constitutional disturbance.

Another cause is frequently found in affections of the lachrymal canal, particularly catarrh of the lachrymal sac and stricture of the duct; in these cases the tears being hindered from flowing through their natural passage into the nose, collect in the eye, flow over the lids and down the cheek; thus the retention of the tears will cause an inflammation of the margins and eventually of the whole structure of the lids. Any other affection which will have the same result (flowing of the tears over the lids), will, of course, produce the same trouble, and this is often found in slight degrees of eversion of the lower lids (ectropion) which displace the puncta lachrymalis, and thus prevent the tears from passing into the sac. In all such cases, the first thing to be done is to open the canaliculus into the sac, and if necessary, the nasal duct into the nose, so as to give a free passage for the tears into that organ, after which the treatment is the same as in uncomplicated cases.

But the most common causes of ciliary blepharitis, are exposure to wind, dust, smoke, etc., especially when complicated with *want of cleanliness;* and it is for this reason we see this trouble so frequently among the poorer classes. And it is upon this point—cleanliness—that the success of our treatment depends to a great extent; so we should impress upon the patient's mind the necessity of it, in terms as forcible as possible.

They should be directed to remove the scales or crusts from the margins of the lids, *as soon as formed*, and not allow them to remain even a few minutes; this should not be done by rubbing, as the patient is inclined to do on account of the itching sensation, for if they do, excoriations are made, lymph is thrown out, and new scabs form, which makes the matter worse than before. But they should be directed to moisten the crusts in warm water, and then carefully remove them with a piece of fine linen, or by drawing the ciliæ between the thumb and fingers; at the same time gentle traction may be made on the lashes, so as to remove all that are loose, as they act only as foreign bodies. Sometimes the scabs are so thick and firm, that moistening in warm water is not sufficient to remove them; in such cases, hot compresses or poultices should be applied for ten or twenty minutes at a time, until they can be easily taken away.

Of the usefulness of external applications there can be no doubt, and without the use of which the cure is often impossible. The remedy that comes nearest being a specific in this disease is Graphites, and the local application of this drug when indicated (in connection with some unguent, as, for example, cosmoline) combined with its internal administration, will be attended with brilliant results, even where the patient and physician have both become discouraged from its persistent, but simply internal administration.

Cosmoline. Many cases have been cured by the use of this substance alone, while in other cases it has been used together with the indicated remedy, with benefit; but very frequently cases come up in which we can obtain no symptoms to base our prescriptions upon; in these cases, cosmoline shows its power. It should be used once or twice a day, or oftener, according to the severity of the case, rubbing a little on the edge of the lids, after they have been properly cleansed. It prevents the forming of new scabs, and the agglutination of the lids, and also seems to exert a beneficial influence over the progress of the disease.

The following prescription has been used by Dr. Liebold with success in many cases:

℞. Liq. Hyd. Nitr., gtts. iii.
Ol. Morrhuæ ℥ii.

In some cases more of the mercury is used, in others less, according to the severity of the symptoms. It is applied in the same way as cosmoline.

Various other ointments and washes have been used with

variable success. But generally we can succeed in the treatment of uncomplicated cases of inflammation of the lids, by careful attention to cleanliness, the external use of a little milk or lard to the lids at night, to prevent their sticking together, and the internal administration of the indicated remedy.

Aconite. Chiefly called for in the acute variety of this trouble especially when caused from *exposure to cold, dry winds. The lids—especially the upper—are red and swollen, with a tight feeling in them, while great heat, dryness burning and sensitiveness to air, are present;* the dry heat is temporarily relieved by cold water. The conjunctiva is usually implicated, when this remedy is called for. Concomitant symptoms of fever, thirst, restlessness, etc., are to be taken into consideration.

Alumina. Chronic inflammation of the lids, (particularly if complicated with granulations) characterized by burning and *dryness* of the lids, especially in the evening; *itching, dryness and excoriation of the canthi. Absence of lachrymation* is very marked. There is usually not much destruction of tissue nor great thickening of the lids.

Apis mel. Chronic blepharitis with thickening of the conjunctival layer, so that the lower lid is everted; also ulceration of the margins of the lids and canthi with *stinging pains*, are reported cured, though we do not think that it is often useful. The *stinging pains* and *œdematous swelling of the lids and conjunctiva*, are the chief local indications.

Argentum nit. *Lids very sore, red and swollen*, especially when complicated with granular conjunctivitis or some other external trouble. There is usually *profuse discharge* from the eyes, causing firm agglutination in the morning. The symptoms are often *relieved in the cold air*, or by cold applications, and may be associated with headache, pain in root of the nose, etc.

Arsenicum. Inflammation of the margins of the lids, which are *thick, red and excoriated by the burning, acrid lachrymation.* (The cheek may also be excoriated.) The lids are sometimes œdematously swollen and spasmodically closed, especially when the cornea is at the same time affected. The *characteristic burn-*

ing pains are important and usually present. The general condition of the patient would influence its selection, as the great restlessness, aggravation after midnight, thirst, etc., so commonly seen in scrofulous children.

Aurum. Rarely useful for uncomplicated blepharitis, except when occurring in scrofulous or syphilitic subjects, after the abuse of Mercury. The lids may be red and ulcerated, with stinging, pricking or itching pain in them. Ciliæ rapidly fall out.

Calc. carb. Blepharitis occurring in persons inclined to grow fat or when found in *unhealthy*, "*pot-bellied*" children of a scrofulous diathesis, who sweat much about the head. The lids are red, swollen and *indurated.* Inflammation of the margins of the lids, causing loss of the eyelashes, with thick, purulent excoriating discharge and burning sticking pains. *Great itching* and burning of the margins of the lids, particularly of the canthi; throbbing pain in the lids. Most of the eye symptoms are worse in the morning, on moving the eyes, and in *damp weather.* Great reliance should be placed on the general cachexia of the patient.

Calc. iodata. Seems to act better than the Carbonate in blepharitis, found in those unhealthy children afflicted with *enlargement of the glands and especially of the tonsils.*

Causticum. Blepharitis, especially when complicated with warts on the eyebrows and lids, and when the symptoms are ameliorated in the open air.

Chamomilla. Of benefit as an intercurrent remedy, even if it does not complete the cure, when found in cross, peevish children, who want to be carried. The local symptoms are not marked.

Cinnabaris. Ciliary blepharitis, with *dull pain over or around the eye.* There may be dryness of the eye or considerable discharge.

Croton tig. When there is complicated with the blepharitis a *vesicular eruption on the lids and face.*

Euphrasia. A valuable remedy when we find the lids red, swollen, excoriated by the profuse, acrid, muco-purulent discharge, and even ulcerated. The *lachrymation is also profuse, acrid and burning*, and often accompanied by fluent coryza. The cheek around the eye is also usually sore and red from the nature of the discharges.

Graphites. This is one of the most important remedies we possess for the chronic form of this disease, though it may be indicated in acute attacks, especially if complicated with ulcers or pustules on the cornea. Particularly useful if the inflammation occurs in scrofulous subjects covered with *eczematous eruptions which are moist, fissured* and bleed easily, situated chiefly on the head and *behind the ears.* Edges of the lids slightly swollen, of a pale red color and covered with *dry scales or scurfs*, or the margins ulcerated. The inflammation may be confined to the canthi, especially the *outer*, *which have a great tendency to crack and bleed upon any attempt to open.* Burning and dryness of the lids are often present, also biting and itching, causing a constant desire to rub them. Important in *eczema of the lids*, if the eruption is moist, and tending to crack while the margins are covered with scales or crusts. We have found excellent results in many cases of blepharitis from the use of grapho-cosmoline as a local application, and strongly recommend its use.

Hepar sulph. Especially adapted to acute phlegmonous inflammation, though may also be useful in certain forms of blepharitis in which the lids are inflamed, sore and corroded, as if eaten out, or if small red swellings are found along the margins of the lids, which are painful in the evening and *upon touch.* There is *general amelioration* from warmth. Often called for when the meibomian glands are affected. For eczema palpebrarum, in which the scabs are thick and honey-comb in character on and around the lids, it is very valuable.

Mercurius sol. Very favorable results have been gained by this remedy in blepharitis, especially if dependent upon or found in a *syphilitic subject*, or if caused from working over *fires or forges. The lids are thick*, *red*, *swollen and ulcerated* (particularly the upper), *and sensitive to heat or cold*, *and to touch. Profuse acrid lachrymation* is usually present, which makes the lids sore, red and painful, especially worse in the open air or by the constant application of cold water. *All the symptoms are worse in the evening after going to bed and from warmth in general;* also from the glare of a fire or any artificial light. The concomitant symptoms should receive special attention, as excoriation of the nose from the acrid coryza, flabby condition of the tongue, nocturnal pains, etc., etc.

Mercurius corr. This form differs very little in its symptomatology from the above, and that is chiefly in degree, *as the pains are generally more severe* and spasmodic in character, *lachrymation more profuse and acrid, secretions thinner and more excoriating*, and inflammatory swelling greater than in any other preparation. Has proved curative in inflammatory swelling of indurated lids, inflammatory swelling of cheeks and parts around the orbits, which are covered with small pustules, and especially in *scrofulous inflammation of the lids.* Nocturnal aggravation of the symptoms is usually present.

Mezereum. Blepharitis accompanied by tinea capitis; or, *eczema of the lids* and head, characterized by *thick hard scabs*, from under which pus exudes on pressure.

Natrum mur. Ciliary blepharitis, particularly if caused by the use of caustics (nitrate of silver). The lids are thick, inflamed, smart and burn, with a feeling of sand in the eye. The lachrymation is acrid, excoriating the lids and cheeks, making them *glossy and shining*, often accompanied by eczema.

Nux vom. Blepharitis ciliaris, with smarting and dryness of the lids, especially *worse in the morning.* Is particularly indicated in ciliary blepharitis dependent upon gastric disturbances.

Petroleum. Has cured many cases of ciliary blepharitis, especially if combined with the use of cosmoline externally. Great reliance should be placed on the occipital headache, rough skin, etc., generally found when this drug is indicated, though has been often used with great advantage when no marked symptoms were present.

Psorinum. Old chronic cases of inflammation of the lids, especially when subject to occasional exacerbations. Has also been of service in the acute variety, when the internal surface of the lids is chiefly affected and there is considerable photophobia. Particularly indicated in a *strumous diathesis*, with unhealthy offensive discharges from the eyes.

Pulsatilla. Blepharitis, both acute and chronic, especially if the glands of the lids are affected (blepharadenitis) or when there is a great tendency to the formation of *styes* or abscesses on the margin of the palpebræ. Blepharitis resulting from high living or fat food, and when accompanied by acne of the face; also in cases in which the tear glands and lachrymal canal are affected. The swelling, redness and discharges vary, though the latter are more often *profuse and bland*, causing agglutination of the lids in the morning. *Itching* and *burning* are the chief sensations experienced. The symptoms are usually *aggravated in the evening*, in a warm room or in a cold draught of air, but *ameliorated in the cool open air.*

Rhus tox. Not often called for in ciliary blepharitis, unless there be *considerable swelling of the lids* and cheek, and profuse lachrymation. Blepharitis resulting from exposure to the wet or worse in damp weather. Its chief use is in acute phlegmonous inflammation of the lids and erysipelas.

Sepia. Both acute and chronic blepharitis, caused by or complicated with uterine disorders. Lids swollen and inflamed, with burning, aching or numb pain in them; also a feeling as if they were too tight and did not cover the ball. *Always worse in the morning and evening.*

Silicea. Blepharitis, with agglutination of the lids in the morning; objects appear as if seen through a fog, ameliorated by wiping the eyes (Euphras.); fluent coryza and corners of the mouth cracked; psoriasis on the arm.

Staphysagria. Blepharitis, in which the margins of the lids are dry, with *hard nodules* on the borders and destruction of the hair follicles.

Sulphur. A remedy called for, especially in the chronic form of this disease, and when found in children of a strumous diathesis, who are irritable and cross by day, and restless and feverish by night; also for blepharitis appearing after the suppression of an eruption or when the patient is covered with eczema. The lids are red, swollen and agglutinated in the morning, or there may be numerous small itching pustules on the margins. The *pains are usually of a sticking character*, though we may have itching, biting, burning, and a variety of other sensations in the lids. There is generally great aversion to water, so that *they cannot bear to have the eyes washed.* Eczematous affections of the lids, like eczema in other portions of the body, which indicate Sulphur, are often controlled.

Tellurium. Eczema of the lids, especially if complicated with a moist eruption behind the ears and *offensive otorrhœa* smelling like fish brine.

Thuya. Tinea ciliaris, dry bran-like eruptions on the lids and fine scales covering the skin generally, eyes weak and suffused in tears.

In addition to the above, the following remedies have also proved serviceable:—Ant. crud., Arg. met., Bell., Clem., Colch., Dig., Kali carb., Lyco., Merc. nitr., Merc. prot., Natrum sulph., Phos. ac., Sang., Seneg., Viola tricol.

ERYSIPELAS OF THE LIDS.

Externally, warm applications should be employed, either dry or moist, as may be most agreeable to the patient. If the chemosis of the conjunctiva be very great, so as to interfere with the nutrition of the cornea, incision of the conjunctiva is thought advisable by some. If pus has formed, a free incision must be made at once to allow it to escape, in order that the scar and contractions of the tissues may be as small as possible. Careful attention must be paid to the general hygienic condition of the patient.

Apis. Erysipelatous inflammation of the lids, with adjacent smooth swelling of the face, especially if the *conjunctiva is chemosed. The upper lid is particularly œdematously swollen and hangs like a sack over the eye.* The photophobia and lachrymation are often very marked. There may be *stinging*, itching, burning or swollen feeling around the eyes and in the brows; also *severe shooting pains* over the eye (right), extending into the ball. The patient may be drowsy, thirstless, etc. (reverse of Arsenicum), and is usually worse in the evening or forepart of the night.

Arsenicum. Erysipelas of the lids, associated with the *general cachectic Arsenic condition*, great prostration, restlessness, thirst, etc. The lids are swollen and œdematous, especially the lower (though mostly non-inflammatory and painless). The pains are of a decided *burning* character, while the aggravations are periodic, but especially after midnight. (Apis before midnight.)

Belladonna. *Lids and surrounding tissues red, swollen and congested*, with throbbing pain in them. The integument may be bright red and shining, though has not the peculiar œdematous look found under Apis and Rhus. *Absence of lachrymation* predominates, in this respect, differing from the other remedies mentioned. The inflammation is no more marked in one lid than in the other. Conjunctiva usually congested. The face is flushed and the headache severe, of a throbbing character.

Rhus tox. Erysipelas of the lids, whether traumatic or not, if there is *much œdematous, erysipelatous swelling of the lids and face, with small watery vesicles scattered over the surface*, and drawing pains in the cheek and head. The lids are usually *spasmodically closed* and upon opening them a *profuse gush of tears takes place.* The conjunctiva is usually chemosed and the aggravation of the symptoms is especially in the latter part of the night and in damp weather. Especially useful if resulting from exposure in the wet, getting the feet wet, or from change in the weather.

Veratrum vir. Dr. Liebold is of the opinion, that this is a valuable remedy for traumatic erysipelas of the lids.

PTOSIS.

This affection is usually complicated with paralysis of one or more of the ocular muscles supplied by the same nerve (oculo-motorius), though frequently only those twigs which supply the levator palpebræ superioris are involved, giving rise to simple drooping of the lid. We rely principally in the treatment upon internal medication, though sometimes *electricity* proves of great value, either used alone or in connection with the indicated remedy. If the disease resists all treatment (dependent upon irremediable causes), operative measures must be resorted to.

Alumina. The upper lids are weak, seem to hang down as if paralyzed, especially the left. *Burning dryness* in the eyes, especially on looking up. *Absence of lachrymation.* Particularly useful for loss of power in the upper lids *met with in old dry cases of granulations.*

Causticum. More benefit has probably been derived from this remedy in the treatment of ptosis than from any other. Its special indication is, *drooping of the lid resulting from the exposure to cold* (Rhus, from damp cold). The symptoms in the proving point very strongly to Caust. as a remedy in this disorder, as, "inclination to close the eyes; they close involuntarily. Sensation of heaviness in the upper lid, as if he could not raise it easily, etc."

Euphrasia. If caused from exposure to cold and wet, and accompanied by catarrhal symptoms of the conjunctiva.

Rhus tox. Especially if found in a *rheumatic diathesis*, and if the result can be traced to *working in the wet, getting the feet damp or to change in the weather.* There may be aching, drawing pains in the head and face, or they may be absent. The concomitant symptoms might point to its selection, though it has proved useful when none are present.

Spigelia. Ptosis, resulting from inflammation or other causes, in which *sharp stabbing pains through the eye* are present. Sometimes hot, scalding lachrymation accompanies the above.

Gelsemium and **Conium** have both been favorably employed in this affection, especially the former, also Lach., Sepia and Veratrum alb. (Comp. paralysis of the muscles.)

TRICHIASIS AND DISTICHIASIS.

The treatment of distorted eyelashes is chiefly surgical, being rarely, if ever, amenable to internal medication. The most common method of dealing with them, if few in number, is to extract them as fast as they grow and become irritating to the eye. Frequent extraction may in time cause the hair bulbs to atrophy, and thus cure the case, though usually this treatment is only palliative. To obtain a permanent cure, operative measures must be resorted to, and a variety of these have been devised and employed with more or less favorable results.

Borax is the only remedy reported to have cured trichiasis, though we have often employed it with no avail.

ENTROPION.

The treatment of inversion of the lids varies according to the cause and duration of the disease. If the entropion is slight and recent, and of spasmodic or senile origin, (especially of the lower lid), a cure may often be effected, by painting the part with *collodion* or by the proper use of adhesive strips. The collodion, however, must be renewed every two or three days or oftener, in order to keep the lid in position. This method will not suffice in an entropion of long duration or considerable degree; in which case we must employ surgical means. A variety of operations have been proposed, though the one most commonly employed is simply the removal of a horizontal fold of integument, parallel and close to the margin of the lid, *including a portion of the orbicularis muscle;* after which the edges of the wound are brought together by three or four sutures. Canthoplasty is frequently beneficial either alone or combined with the previous operation.

Remedies may be useful if the inversion is recent and only slight in degree.

Aconite. If acute and accompanied by inflammatory symptoms, dryness, burning, etc.

Calcarea. Cases are reported cured, especially the senile form.

Natrum mur. Entropion following the use of caustics for granular lids, (particularly nitrate of silver).

ECTROPION.

In acute cases of eversion of the lids, consequent upon inflammation and hypertrophy of the conjunctiva, they should be replaced and retained in position for several days by the use of a compress bandage. This bandage properly and patiently applied is frequently all that is necessary. Scarification or cauterization of the hypertrophied conjunctiva has been advised in acute cases, if the bandage alone is not all that is required.

Narrowing the palpebral fissure (tarsoraphia) may be useful in both the acute and chronic stages of the disease.

The operations, to which we must often resort, recommended for this affection, are legion, and must necessarily vary in nearly every case, according to the cause, degree and position of the eversion.

Apis. Is especially indicated in the first stage of this affection, in which the swelling is very great.

Argent. nit. If the lids are swollen, inflamed, everted and the *puncta lachrymalia very red and prominent.* The discharge of tears and pus is marked.

Hamamelis virg. A dilute solution of "Pond's Extract" applied locally is said to have cured a case, occurring during the course of a severe conjunctivitis.

Nitric acid. Relief of ectropion is reported to have been obtained.

We place little reliance upon internal medication in either entropion or ectropion, believing that, (except in the first stage) the knife must usually be employed.

LUPUS AND EPITHELIOMA.

Cases of malignant tumor are reported to have been cured by our remedies, though owing, probably, to our limited knowledge, many cases are met that prove very obstinate to internal medication. We, therefore, would advise *excision*, if the disease is circumscribed and moderate in extent; care being taken that all the morbid tissue is removed. The edges of the wound may be brought together by sutures, or a plastic operation may be made, bringing the integument from the temple or some adjoining point.

Various caustics have also been employed, chief among which may be mentioned, caustic potash, nitrate of silver, chloride of zinc, arsenic paste, acetic acid, etc.

Dr. Althaus advises electrolysis.

If the disease is very extensive, involving the tissues of the face to any extent so that extirpation is impracticable, we then rely chiefly upon our internal remedies, using only such local applications as prove agreeable, and of temporary relief to the patient. For instance, if the discharge is profuse and offensive, a weak solution of carbolic acid, salicylic acid, or some other disinfectant proves of service. An application from which we have often seen excellent results, is carbolic acid and linseed oil (four grains to the ounce); it relieves the patient and sometimes seems to exert a beneficial effect over the progress of the disease.

Apis. Lupus non exedens, *sharp stinging pains* and tendency towards puffiness of the lower lid.

Hydrocotyle asiatica. Has obtained a high reputation in the hands of Dr. Boileau as a remedy for lupus, and deserves our attention. (We have, however, failed to perceive any results from its use.)

Phytolacca dec. Benefit seems to have been derived in relieving, if not curing malignant ulcers of the lids, when used both externally and internally.

Lycopodium. Has been followed by favorable results in lupus.

HORDEOLUM.

We are not often called upon to prescribe for a single stye, but usually to prevent the occurrence of frequent crops. If we do see the case at its very outset, cold compresses may be used with advantage, though usually more benefit is derived, especially after its commencement, from hot poultices. If pus has formed, as shown by a yellow point, a small incision can be made to permit its ready escape. If dependent, as it frequently is, upon any impairment of the general health, proper hygienic measures must be advised.

Graphites. Useful in preventing the recurrence of styes. (Compare general symptoms of patient.)

Hepar. If suppuration has already commenced and there is throbbing pain, great sensitiveness to touch and amelioration by warmth.

Pulsatilla. This is an excellent remedy for styes of every description and in every stage of the disease. If given early before the formation of pus, it will often cause them to abort; if used later, relief from the pain and hastening of the process of cure is frequently produced, while, as a remedy for the prevention of the recurrence of successive crops, it is surpassed by none. Is especially useful if *dependent upon some gastric derangement*, as from indulgence in high living, fat food, etc., and if *accompanied by acne of the face;* also when found in amenorrhœic females or the peculiar Pulsatilla temperament.

Staphysagria. Recurrence of styes, especially on the lower lid, which are inclined to abort and leave little hard nodules on the lid.

Sulphur. To prevent the constant recurrence of successive crops, especially if occurring in a strumous diathesis, showing itself by eruptions, boils, etc., in various portions of the body. Cannot bear to have the eyes washed, and is restless and feverish at night.

Thuya. Obstinate forms of styes, which seem to resist treatment and form little hard nodules on the margins of the lids.

The following remedies have also been recommended and

used with advantage:—Acon., Alum., Ambr., Ars., Calc., Canth., Caust., Colch., Colocy., Con., Dig., Electricity, Ferr., Lyco., Menyan., Merc., Nat. mur., Phos. ac., Phos., Rhus, Seneg., Stann. and Valerian.

TUMORS OF THE LID.

(*Chalazion, verucœ, sebaceous, fibroid, fatty, etc.*)

Tarsal tumors are, as a rule, immediately subjected to the knife by the old school, and no doubt in the case of a single tumor, this is the quickest way of curing. The treatment of cystic tumors by a seton through the tumor, is recommended in some cases.

If the patient objects to the use of the knife, or if there be many tumors on the lids, we may depend upon our homœopathic remedies which have so often proved serviceable.

Calc. carb. Has often proved valuable in tarsal tumors occurring in fat, flabby subjects.

Causticum. Tumors, especially warts found on the lids and eyebrows.

Conium. Indurations of the lids remaining after inflammation.

Hepar. Tarsal tumors that have become inflamed and are sensitive to touch.

Nitric acid. If of syphilitic origin or dependent upon the abuse of mercury. Condyloma on the lower lid, suppurating and bleeding easily; profuse hot lachrymation; cheek around swollen and inflamed, with burning, sticking pains.

Pulsatilla. Tarsal tumors of recent origin, that are subject to inflammation or are accompanied by catarrhal conditions of the eye. The temperament and general symptoms will decide us.

Sepia. Tumors resulting from styes are said to have been caused to disappear.

Silicea. Favorable results have been obtained in cystic tumors and in a tendency to suppuration.

Staphysagria. An important remedy for tumors of the lid. Enlargement of the glands of the lids, which are red and accompanied by tensive, tearing pains, especially in the evening. Little *indurations of the lids resulting from styes* or if successive crops of small tarsal tumors are constantly recurring, this drug would be especially indicated.

Thuya. This is another of our chief remedies for tarsal tumors, whether single or multiple, especially if they appear like a condyloma either on the internal or external surface of the lid. We have seen them disappear by simply giving the drug internally, though it often seems to act better, if we use, at the same time, the tincture externally. Is also recommended for the prevention of their return after removal by the knife. For condylomata or warty excrescences on the lids, especially if occurring in syphilitic subjects, this drug deserves attention.

Baryta carb. and jod., Graph., Lyco., Kali brom. and jod., Merc., Teuc., and Sulph. may be tried.

INJURIES OF THE LIDS.

Immediately after a contused wound of the lids, cold compresses should be employed; they should be applied with a firm bandage, which often proves of advantage in limiting the amount of ecchymosis.

Arnica, our great remedy for all contusions, deserves its extensive reputation for curing "black eyes," as there is no other drug better adapted to this condition. A solution of the tincture in water, ten drops to the ounce, is usually employed, though both stronger and weaker solutions are in vogue.

Incised wounds are generally more serious in nature, though vary greatly according to situation, both in danger and results of treatment. The first object in view should be to bring together the edges of the wound by means of sutures, adhesive strips or collodion; after which the application of a solution of Calendula, ten drops to the ounce of water, should be applied. If the tissues are very much bruised, Arnica may be applied, though as a rule Calendula will be found more useful in cut wounds.

Hamamelis and Ledum have both been recommended for wounds of the lids.

Burns and scalds must be treated as usual in other parts of the body, except that care should be taken to prevent the union of the lids (anchyloblepharon) by frequently opening them, and by inunction of the edges with simple cerate, cosmoline, etc. Also great attention should be paid to the prevention of a cicatrix (which will cause ectropion), by keeping the skin on the stretch, by bandage, etc., during the period of cicatrization. Cosmoline is especially recommended as an external application.

When dependent upon stings of insects, the sting should be removed and cold water dressings applied.

ANCHYLOBLEPHARON.

The union between the edges of the lids are to be divided by a scalpel and then prevented from uniting by the use of oil and frequent opening of the lids.

CONGENITAL MALFORMATIONS.

Congenital malformations, as epicanthus, coloboma, etc., are only to be remedied by the use of the knife.

CONJUNCTIVA.

CONJUNCTIVITIS CATARRHALIS, ACUTE AND CHRONIC.

The first point in the treatment should be the removal of any exciting cause. To accomplish this, the lids should first be everted and examined for the presence of a foreign body, which, if detected, should be removed. Should the conjunctivitis depend upon any anomaly of refraction, this should be corrected. If due to straining of the eyes in reading, writing, etc. (especially in the evening), or to exposure to wind, dust, or any bright light, as working over a fire; directions to abstain from overuse, or to protect the eyes from the injurious causes, should be given. Should the case be very severe, the patient may be confined to his room, though this is rarely required in pleasant weather. As a local remedy, cold applications are especially recommended: but care should be taken that they are not employed too constantly, particularly if there is œdema of the lids, when they often prove harmful. Great reliance should be placed upon the sensations experienced by the patient, regarding the use of warm or cold applications, as the beneficial results obtained vary in different cases. Sometimes the same remedy that we employ internally is used with benefit externally. Cleanliness should be especially required. To prevent the formation of crusts on the lids, the edges may be smeared at night with a little vaseline, simple cerate, cream or the like. Astringents, such as sulphate of zinc or copper, or nitrate of silver are chiefly relied upon by the old school, though not advised until after the acute symptoms have subsided. Atropine should not be used unless there be iritic complication.

The attendants should be warned that the discharge is contagious, and that the sponges, towels, etc., used upon the patient, should not be employed for any other purpose.

Aconite. Is especially indicated in the *first stage of catarrhal* *inflammation* prior to exudation, when the conjunctiva is intensely hyperæmic and chemosed, with severe pain in the eye, often so terrible that one wishes to die; or, as is frequently the case, only a feeling of *burning and general heat in the eye, with great dryness;* there may also be an aching or bruised pain, or a feeling as if the ball were enlarged and protruding, making the lids tense. The eye is generally very sensitive, especially to air. This is the first remedy to be thought of for conjunctivitis dependent upon *exposure to cold, dry air.*

For inflammatory conditions of the conjunctiva, resulting from the *irritant action of foreign bodies* in that tissue, there is no better remedy.

Allium cepa. Of use in acute catarrhal conjunctivitis, associated with a similar condition of the air passages; the lachrymation is scalding, profuse and not excoriating, though the nasal discharge is so (reverse of Euphrasia).

Apis mel. Especially called for in the acute form of conjunctivitis, when the conjunctiva is bright red and puffy, lachrymation hot and moderately profuse, and pains in the eye, burning, biting or *stinging;* sometimes the pains are very severe, darting through the eye, or possibly around the eye and in the brows. Photophobia may be present. The *œdematous condition of the lids*, especially the upper, which is usually present in the cases in which Apis is indicated, is an important symptom. There is, generally, aggravation in the evening and fore part of the night. Although the lachrymation is hot and burning, yet it does not excoriate the lids, as in cases in which Arsenicum is indicated. General symptoms of dropsy, absence of thirst, etc., would suggest this remedy to our minds.

Argentum nit. Should be employed if the *discharge becomes profuse*, apparently taking the character of purulent ophthalmia. It may also be indicated in the chronic form of conjunctivitis, when the conjunctiva is scarlet red and the papillæ hypertrophied. The inflammatory symptoms usually subside in the open air, and are aggravated in a warm room.

Arnica. In conjunctivitis resulting from blows and various injuries Arnica is often beneficial.

Arsenicum. Occasionally useful in acute conjunctivitis marked by chemosis of the conjunctiva, much hot, scalding lachrymation, *burning pains, especially at night*, and œdematous condition of the lids, particularly the lower lid. It is also indicated in the chronic form when the *lachrymation and discharge from the eyes are acrid*, excoriating the lids and cheek, the balls burn as if on fire, especially at night. Warm applications generally relieve. The attacks of inflammation are frequently periodic in occurrence and often alternate from one eye to the other.

Belladonna. The remedy in the early stages of catarrhal conjunctivitis, when there is great dryness of the eyes, with a sense of dryness and stiffness in the thickened red lids, and smarting, burning pains in the eyes. Photophobia is often marked. Much dependence should be placed, however, upon the concomitant symptoms of headache, red face, etc., etc. It will be seen that Bell. is similar to Aconite and that both correspond to the early stages of the disease. The dryness of the eyes exists equally under both drugs; but under Acon. we have much more heat and burning in and around the eye than under Bell.

Calcarea carb. Occasionally useful in catarrhal conjunctivitis *caused by working in water.*

Chamomilla. Catarrhal conjunctivitis, occurring in peevish children during dentition. Conjunctiva so congested, that blood oozes out.

Cinnabaris. May be called for in conjunctivitis, especially with the characteristic symptom of *pain above the eye, extending from the internal to the external canthus*, (usually above, though sometimes below).

Euphrasia. In this drug, we have a very valuable remedy for both acute and chronic catarrhal conjunctivitis, especially acute. It is useful in catarrhal inflammation of the eye, caused by exposure to the cold and also in that of the eyes and nose found in the first stage of measles. In the selection of this drug, we are guided chiefly by the objective symptoms as the subjective are not very definite, there being a variety of different sensations. The conjunctiva is intensely red, even to chemosis. The *lachrymation is profuse, acrid, burning, while the discharge from the eye, which is also quite profuse, is thick, yellow, muco-purulent and acrid, making the lids and cheek sore and excoriated.* (The secretion is also excoriating under Arsenic and Mercurius, but is thinner.) *Blurring of the vision relieved by winking*, dependent upon the secretion covering the cornea temporarily, is especially characteristic of this remedy.

Graphites. Sometimes indicated, especially in the chronic form of catarrhal conjunctivitis, though it is more particularly the remedy for phlyctenular ophthalmia. The redness, photophobia and lachrymation are usually well marked, but may vary to a great extent. The discharges from the eye, if present, are thin and acrid, while the nose is sore, excoriated and often surrounded by thick, moist scabs. Dry scurfs are frequently found on the lids, while the *external canthi crack and bleed easily.*

Hepar sulph. Another remedy more useful in strumous ophthalmia; though it is sometimes employed with benefit in the catarrhal form, as when the conjunctiva is much congested even to chemosis, with considerable photophobia and lachrymation, while the lids are much swollen and very sensitive to touch. The discharge is of a muco-purulent character and often well marked. The pains are throbbing, aching or lancinating and relieved by warmth, so that one wishes to keep the eye covered most of the time.

Ignatia. Has been successfully used in catarrhal ophthalmia, especially in nervous hysterical subjects, consequent upon traumatic or other causes, when there is a sensation as if a grain of sand were rolling around under the lid, with great dryness, and lachrymation only when exposed to the sunlight.

Merc. sol. In Mercury, we possess an important remedy for catarrhal conjunctivitis, and this preparation is most commonly required, though some other may be employed, if the concomitant symptoms so indicate. The redness and dread of light are usually well marked, especially in the evening, by artificial light. The *lachrymation is profuse, burning and excoriating, and the muco-purulent discharges thin and acrid*, making the lids and cheek red and sore. The pains vary in character and are not confined to the eye, but extend into the forehead and temples, are *always worse at night* especially before midnight, in extreme heat or cold and in damp weather, and are often temporarily ameliorated by cold water. It is especially indicated in syphilitic subjects, and when the concomitant symptoms of soreness of the head, excoriation of the nose, nocturnal pains, etc., etc., are present.

Nux vomica. Is not very often called for in this variety of conjunctivitis. It would be suggested to our minds if there were much dread of light, marked *morning aggravation* and accompanying gastric symptoms. Hartmann and Altschul highly recommend its use in conjunctivitis, when there is great tendency to hemorrhage.

Pulsatilla. This is another of our standard remedies for catarrhal conjunctivitis, especially the acute form, though it is also useful in the chronic. It is particularly to be thought of in conjunctivitis occurring in the colored race, as well as in the mild, tearful female. Catarrhal inflammations resulting from a cold, an attack of measles, traumatic and various other causes, have been benefited. The redness is variable and may even amount to chemosis. The pains in the eye, are burning, itching or lancinating, usually worse in the evening, when in the wind, and after reading, but relieved by the cool open air. The lachrymation is often profuse by day with a purulent discharge at night; though, generally, a *moderately profuse mucopurulent discharge of a white color and bland character*, which agglutinates the lids in the morning, is to be found. Gastric and other concomitant symptoms if present will influence our choice.

Rhus tox. Is the chief remedy for conjunctivitis caused by *exposure to the wet* (Calc.), especially when the conjunctiva is much chemosed, with some photophobia, *profuse lachrymation* and *œdematous swelling of the lids.* A rheumatic diathesis would especially suggest this remedy.

Sanguinaria. Benefit has been derived from its use in catarrhal conditions of the conjunctiva with burning in the edges of the lids, worse in the afternoon, or when the affection is dependent upon stricture of the lachrymal duct.

Sepia. Acute catarrhal conjunctivitis, with drawing sensation in the external canthi and smarting in the eyes, ameliorated by bathing in cold water, and *aggravated morning and evening;* and conjunctivitis, with muco-purulent discharge from the eyes in the morning and great dryness in the evening, have been speedily relieved by Sepia. It is frequently found useful in inflammatory affections of the conjunctiva of an asthenic character, the conjunctiva exhibiting a dull, red color, with some photophobia and swelling of the lids, especially in the morning.

Spigelia. Rarely useful, though, according to Lippe, it has benefited a case occurring in the left eye, with *severe lancinating pains* in the eye and left temple, worse at night, preventing sleep.

Sulphur. This is one of our chief remedies in both the acute and chronic forms of catarrhal conjunctivitis. The degree of redness may vary greatly; it may be confined to one eye or may involve both. The lids may be swollen or remain unaffected. The *sharp, darting pains, like pins piercing the eye,* occurring at any time of the day or night, will furnish our chief indication. A severe pain darting through the eye back into the head, from 1 to 3 A.M., waking the patient from sleep, is also an important indication. A variety of other sensations may be present; as pressing, tensive, cutting or burning pains, a feeling of sand in the eyes, etc. The patients are usually *feverish and restless at night.*

Zincum. Has been useful in conjunctivitis, especially when confined to the *inner half of the eye,* (usually without photophobia) with much discharge; worse towards evening and in the cool air. Generally there is itching, and perhaps pain, in the internal canthus.

The following remedies have also been used with benefit or may be indicated in occasional cases:—Alumina, Chelidonium, Chloral, Crocus, Cuprum al., Cuprum sulph., Digitalis, Euphorbium, Eupatorium perf., Kali bichr., Natrum mur., Senega, Silicea and Thuya.

CONJUNCTIVITIS PURULENTA.

Under this head we shall include gonorrhœal ophthalmia and ophthalmia neonatorum, which are only different forms of purulent conjunctivitis. If the attack is very severe, the patient may be confined to a darkened room, or even to bed; if only one eye is affected, the other should be kept closed, in order to prevent any of the matter coming in contact with this eye, for the discharge is very contagious, especially in the gonorrhœal form and in that found in new-born children. On this account great care should be exercised, both by the nurse and physician, to protect their own eyes and those of others by providing that the sponges, towels, etc., are used only by the patient, and also that their hands are thoroughly cleansed before touching another eye, for often the physician and other patients have been inoculated and vision destroyed through carelessness on this point. Fresh air and nourishing diet are important aids to treatment. But the special and primary point to be attended to in the treatment is *cleanliness*. To ensure this, the discharges should be often removed by dropping tepid warm water into the inner canthus, until all the pus has been washed away or by cleansing with the palpebral syringe. This should be done at intervals of from fifteen minutes to an hour during the day and occasionally through the night, according to the severity of the case. The old school rely chiefly upon the use of astringents: sulphate of copper and zinc and the nitrate of silver; the latter being the favorite remedy.

When the cornea becomes ulcerated, some operative measures or the use of atropine, may be required; but as this is a complication, we will not dwell upon it. Canthoplasty might be necessary to relieve the pressure upon the eyeball, if the lids were much swollen and very tense.

Aconite. May be indicated in the very first stage, according to the symptoms given under catarrhal conjunctivitis; but it will be found of little or no avail after the purulent discharge has once appeared.

Apis mel. Is useful in violent cases of purulent conjunctivitis and ophthalmia neonatorum, when there is *great swelling (œdematous) of the lids and adjacent cellular tissue.* The conjunctiva is also congested, puffy, chemosed, and full of dark, red veins. The discharge is moderate, not profuse, though the lachrymation is well marked. The character of the pains, which are *stinging and shooting*, is an important indication. There is usually much photophobia accompanying the hot lachrymation (Rhus). The symptoms are aggravated in the evening. Objectively, the Rhus cases are similar to Apis; the character of the pains will usually serve to distinguish between the two.

Argentum nit. This is the remedy, *par excellence*, for all forms of purulent ophthalmia. We have witnessed the most intense chemosis with strangulated vessels, most profuse purulent discharge and commencing haziness of cornea with a tendency to slough, subside rapidly under this remedy, internally administered. We believe there is no need of cauterization; but that all the beneficial results may be obtained by its use in the potencies. The subjective symptoms are almost none. Their very absence, with the profuse purulent discharge and the swollen lids, swollen from being distended by a collection of pus in the eye or from swelling of the sub-conjunctival tissues and not from infiltration of the connective tissue of the lids themselves (as in Rhus or Apis) indicates the drug.

By its employment as a cauterizating agent, as used by the Old School, there is no doubt that many cases of purulent conjunctivitis are cured, though with risk to the cornea, as is attested by the results of this treatment. These sad results, viz.: perforation of cornea, dense leucoma, etc., we claim are, to a great extent, averted by the use of the remedy in the potencies, either internally alone or both internally and externally. We are in the habit of using the thirtieth potency internally, and, at the same time, a solution of five or ten grains to two drams of water of the first, third or thirtieth dilution as an external application, all the time taking great care to ensure cleanliness; and we have yet to see the first case go on to destruction of the cornea. Of course this remedy will not cure every case, though it will the majority, when simply purulent, gonorrhœal, or of that form found in new-born children.

Calcarea carb. The discharges from the eye, under this drug, are often profuse and therefore it has been used with advantage in some cases of purulent or infantile ophthalmia, characterized by profuse, yellowish-white discharge, œdema of the lids and ulceration of the cornea. It is, however, especially useful for the *results* of purulent ophthalmia, clearing up the opacities of the cornea, etc.

It is specially indicated when the trouble arises from working in the water. In the selection of this drug, great reliance should be placed upon the general condition (cachexia) of the patient, as the eye symptoms are not very characteristic.

Chamomilla. Is often of great service in ophthalmia neonatorum as an intercurrent remedy, even if it does not remove the whole trouble, which it frequently does. It is indicated when the child is very fretful and wants to be carried all the time and when the usual symptoms of the disease are present even though the cornea has been invaded. Sometimes the conjunctiva is so much congested that blood may ooze out, drop by drop, from between the swollen lids, especially upon any attempt to open them (Nux).

Chelidonium. Buchmann reports a case of severe inflammation of the eye, occurring in a man 62 years of age, caused by getting the feet wet, and which was cured with Chelidonium^{6}. The lids were thick, red, swollen and the lashes partially absent; conjunctiva swollen and dark red; thick, yellow discharge from the eyes; agglutination in the mornings and great photophobia, with burning, darting pains in the eyes.

Chlorine. Aqua chlorata as an external application, has proved a very valuable remedy in the various forms of purulent ophthalmia. Cases have been relieved by it when used alone, as well as with the indicated remedy given at the same time internally (which has generally been the case). The strong solution is sometimes employed, though we usually dilute it to one-half, one-third or still weaker.

Euphrasia. Is useful, especially in that form found in new-born children, more often in the later stages of the disease than at the beginning, as can well be understood by examining the symptoms already given under catarrhal conjunctivitis, where the indications have been stated.

Hepar sulph. May be indicated in any form of this disease, particularly when the cornea has become implicated and ulceration has taken place. The *lids may be swollen, spasmodically closed, bleeding easily upon any attempt to open them and very sensitive to touch.* The conjunctiva is much reddened, *chemosed* and the *discharge is considerable* and of a yellowish-white color. The *photophobia is intense*, lachrymation profuse and pain severe, of a throbbing, aching character and relieved by warmth; any draught of air aggravating the symptoms. When the *ulceration is severe* and *hypopion* has taken place, Hepar is especially the remedy.

Kreosote. Blennorrhœa of the conjunctiva when the discharge is moderately profuse and marked by much smarting in the eyes.

Mercurius. Has been employed with benefit, particularly in ophthalmia neonatorum when the *discharges are thin and excoriating and caused by syphilitic leucorrhœa.* It is also one of our best remedies for gonorrhœal ophthalmia and for purulent conjunctivitis found in syphilitic subjects, whether it be acquired or hereditary. The discharge, as has been said, is thin and excoriating, making the lids and cheek sore and raw. The lachrymation and photophobia are usually marked and the pains severe, though variable in character and always worse at night. Is more commonly called for in the later stage of the disease and especially if the cornea has become involved. The concomitant symptoms are important aids in the selection. Mercurius corr., Mercurius sol. and Mercurius prec. ruber have all been successfully used, though the eye symptoms, we believe, vary little in these preparations, except perhaps being more intense under the corrosivus.

Nitric acid. Is especially advised for gonorrhœal ophthalmia. Much benefit has been derived from its employment in this affection. Lids much swollen, red, hard and painful, conjunctiva hyperæmic and chemosed, cornea dim, great photophobia and lachrymation and copious discharge of yellow pus, which flows down the cheek, pressing and burning pain in the eye worse at night. The cheeks are also usually much swollen and painful.

Pulsatilla. This remedy stands high in the treatment of purulent conjunctivitis, when the *discharge is profuse and bland.* Benefit has been gained from its use in blennorrhœa of the conjunctiva, caused by the gonorrhœal contagion. It is however most frequently useful in ophthalmia neonatorum, characterized by the usual well-marked symptoms. Many cases of this form of conjunctivitis have been cured by this drug alone, though we believe that it is particularly called for, as an intercurrent remedy, during the treatment by Argent. nit.; for, often when the improvement under the latter remedy is at a stand still, a few doses of Pulsatilla will materially hasten the progress of the cure. The symptoms are usually worse in the evening and ameliorated in the open air.

Rhus tox. Has been employed with great benefit in this form of conjunctivitis, though it is particularly recommended by Hartmann, Garay and others for ophthalmia neonatorum. When the trouble arises from *exposure to the wet* this remedy suggests itself. The *lids are red*, *œdematous* and spasmodically closed. The palpebral conjunctiva is especially inflamed, so that when the lids are opened a thick, red swelling appears, with a *copious*, *thick*, *yellow*, *purulent discharge*, or the discharge may be less and a *profuse gush of tears takes place.* The child is usually cachectic, restless and its head hot. It has been used both externally and internally.

Sulphur. Is not so useful in this variety of conjunctivitis, as in the pustular or even the catarrhal form, though it has been of service more frequently in that form found in newborn children, especially when the trouble has become chronic and when not dependent upon syphilis. The symptoms observed are not characteristic, with the exception, perhaps, of the sharp sticking pains, as if pins were sticking in the eye.

We rely, to a great extent, in selecting this drug, upon the general condition (scrofulous cachexia) of the patient.

Tartar emet. Rosenberg reports a case of severe obstinate gonorrhœal ophthalmia cured, though the urethral discharge was increased by the use of this remedy.

Other remedies, as Con., Cup. al., Cup. sulph., Dulc., Lyc., Natrum mur., and Nux vomica have been successfully employed.

CONJUNCTIVITIS TRACHOMATOSA, ACUTE AND CHRONIC.

(With or without pannus.)

As this form of conjunctivitis is usually found among the lower classes, or those who are constantly exposed to wind and dust, care should be taken that these exciting causes be removed as far as possible, cleanliness and proper hygienic measures being very important aids in the treatment of this affection.

It should be remembered that the discharges from granular lids are especially contagious, and that whole families or a whole school may be inoculated from one member, by an indiscriminate use of towels, etc.; therefore strict attention should be paid to the prevention of its extension.

There is no reason why trachoma should not be cured by the internal administration of medicines alone, but owing to the present inadequate knowledge of our drugs in this affection, a majority of the cases we meet, prove so extremely obstinate to treatment, that both the patient and doctor become discouraged. If a cure can be effected by internal medication, it is much more permanent and better for the patient, than if total reliance is placed upon local applications; but we would not hesitate to use local remedies if there was no particular indication for any special drug, or if the case proved very obstinate. In addition to the external application to be found below, we would also recommend tannic acid and glycerine, about ten grains to the ounce, especially in trachoma complicated with pannus. In acute aggravations of granular lids, the use of ice bags to the eye often proves very agreeable to the patient, and seems to control the intensity of the inflammatory process.

Aconite. In the first stage of granular conjunctivitis, when the eyes are inflamed, hot, dry, burning and very painful, Aconite should be given; also in *acute aggravation of granulated lids and pannus*, with excessive hyperæmia, heat and dryness, especially if the aggravation be induced by over-heating from violent exercise or by exposure to dry, cold air.

Alumen exsiccatum. This remedy, first suggested, we believe by Dr. Liebold, is of great value in all forms of trachoma, whether complicated with pannus or not. It is employed by dusting the crude powder on the inner surface of the lids, allowing it to remain about a minute and then washing it off with pure water, and at the same time giving the lower preparations internally.

Alumina. Cases of chronic granular lids frequently yield to this drug, when there is marked dryness of the lids and eye, especially in the evening, with burning, itching and pressure in the eyes; agglutination mornings; the upper lids are weak, and seem to hang down as if paralyzed. The symptoms of loss of power in the upper lids are often met with in old dry cases of granulation; in these cases Alumina does good.

Argentum nit. Especially serviceable in the early stages of acute granular conjunctivitis, when the conjunctiva is intensely pink or scarlet red, and the *discharge is profuse* and inclined to be muco-purulent.

Arsenicum. Indicated in chronic granular lids, when the palpebral conjunctiva only is inflamed; the lids are painful, dry and rub against the ball; they burn and can scarcely be opened. Chiefly called for, however, when the pains are intense, burning and the lachrymation very excoriating.

Aurum met. Is the appropriate remedy for many cases of trachoma, either with or without pannus (especially however, when pannus is present); there is probably no other remedy which has only been employed internally, that has cured more cases. We therefore highly recommend its use, though the local symptoms which lead us to its selection, have not yet been found peculiar or characteristic. The pains may be burning or dull in character, compelling the patient to close the lids. They are usually worse in the morning and ameliorated by the application of cold water. For the corneal ulcerations found in pannus, Aurum is of great value.

The Muriate of gold is frequently employed, though the symptoms, as far as known, vary but slightly from those of the metal.

Belladonna. As a temporary remedy in acute aggravations of granular lids, may be beneficial; as when, after taking cold, the eyes become sensitive to air and light, with dryness and a gritty feeling.

Calcarea carb. Conjunctivitis trachomatosa with pannus, caused by working in the water, with much redness and lachrymation, has been relieved by this drug. The general condition of the patient will, to a great extent, lead to its selection.

Chinium mur. Marked improvement has been observed from the internal use of this drug in trachoma, with and without pannus.

Cuprum al. The aluminate of copper has been successfully used to a great extent in trachoma, either with or without pannus. The results obtained are usually much more satisfactory than those from the sulphate of copper, which is the main reliance of the old school in the treatment of this disorder. It is employed locally by application of the crystals to the granulations, at the same time giving the remedy in the potencies internally.

Euphrasia. Trachoma, with or without pannus, if the eye is very red and irritable, with *profuse lachrymation* and *thick discharge*, which *excoriates the lids and cheek.*

Kali bich. Trachoma with pannus; much discharge; everything appears slightly red; usually not much photophobia or redness of conjunctiva, though ulceration of the cornea may be present; eyes seem to feel better when lying on the face.

Mercurius praec. rub. In trachoma with pannus, it is a valuable remedy; rarely of much use in acute cases, but especially adapted to old chronic cases, when the cornea is covered with pannus of a high degree, with considerable redness, discharge and photophobia. The granulations may be present or may have been already removed by caustics.

Mercurius protoiod. Especially if pannus accompanies the trachoma, and the eye is quite red and painful, with photophobia and acrid discharges, tongue coated yellow at the base. Is the remedy for *ulceration of a pannoused cornea, particularly if superficial.*

Natrum mur. Particularly useful in chronic cases and when the lids have been already treated by caustics (especially the nitrate of silver). The pannus or the irritable condition of the eye, resulting from or kept up by the scarred palpebral conjunctiva found after cauterization, is often greatly relieved by this drug. The lachrymation is acrid and excoriating, as well as the discharges which are thin, watery, and make the cheek raw and sore. The pains are variable, though sometimes we have a sharp pain over the eye upon looking down, which is very marked. The skin of the face round the eye, is often glossy and shining.

Natrum phos. Granular conjunctivitis, where the granulations appear like small blisters, (Thuya).

Nux vom. Of service in old cases of trachoma that have had much treatment, especially when complicated with pannus. Nux is frequently of great benefit in commencing the treatment of granular lids, with or without pannus; also as an intercurrent remedy, for the morning aggravation is particularly marked under this drug and in the disease. It will rarely however, effect a cure, unassisted by any other remedy.

Petroleum. Valuable in granular conjunctivitis with pannus, especially when occurring in a scrofulous habit with considerable white discharge from the eye, roughness of the cheek, occipital headache, etc.

Pulsatilla. Chiefly adapted to trachoma, uncomplicated with pannus, occurring in anæmic amenorrhœic females. The granulations are generally very fine (papillary trachoma); the eye is sometimes dry or there may be excessive secretion of bland mucus. There may also be soreness of the ball to touch, and itching or pain in the eye, which is worse in the evening, and better in the cool air or by cold applications.

Rhus tox. Is frequently of use in relieving the intensity of the symptoms found in conjunctivitis granulosa with pannus. The eye is quite red, with much photophobia and profuse lachrymation. No remedy acts so powerfully as Rhus tox. in diminishing the profuse secretion of tears.

Sulphur. Trachoma, acute and chronic, with and without pannus, has been benefited by this drug and is often called for as an intercurrent remedy, even if it does not complete the cure alone. It is especially indicated when the *pains are sharp and lancinating* in character, and worse in the morning; and when the lids are glued together by the secretion during the night. The application of water is not agreeable to the patient and it often aggravates the disease.

Thuya occid. Favorable results have been gained by the use of this remedy in conjunctivitis trachomatosa, when the granulations were large, like warts or blisters, with burning in the lids and eyes, worse at night; photophobia by day, and suffusion of the eyes in tears.

The following remedies have also been employed with favorable results:—Causticum, Chin. tan., Cinnabaris, Conium, Cupr. sulph., Hepar, Mercurius, Sepia, Tartar emet. and Zinc.

OPHTHALMIA PHLYCTENULARIS.

(Syn., Ophthalmia scrofulosa, Ophthalmia exanthem., Keratitis phlyct., Conjunctivitis phlyct., etc.)

We have thought best to include under this head the various forms of pustular inflammation of the eye, whether affecting the cornea or conjunctiva, as the etiology, symptomatology, course and treatment vary little in either case; in fact those remedies which have been found useful when the cornea is invaded, are also our chief reliance in this form of inflammation of the conjunctiva.

The first points to be attended to are cleanliness and regulation of diet. The eyes should be bathed often in luke-warm water, and any little scabs which have formed on the lids immediately removed, as they only prove a source of irritation. If there is considerable photophobia and the child rubs the eye much, a compress bandage will prevent this, and, at the same time, by keeping the lids closed, will relieve the irritation to the eyeball, occasioned by their constant opening and closing; it also excludes the light, relieving the photophobia, soaks up the tears and so prevents their running over the cheek, making it sore and excoriated. The bandage if used, though it is not commonly necessary, should be removed every four or five hours and the eyes cleansed. External applications should not, as a rule, be employed, as we can usually cure better and quicker with internal remedies alone, if we are careful in the selection of our drugs, although sometimes they may be useful and necessary; thus, occasionally a case will be found which has proved very obstinate to treatment, ciliary injection great, photophobia intense and pupil a little sluggish—where a weak solution of atropine dropped into the eye, once or twice a day, will be of great benefit.

Apis mel. Pustular keratitis with dark chemosed conjunctiva and swollen lids (œdematous). This puffy condition of the conjunctiva and lids is very important, especially when accompanied by burning, *stinging* or shooting pains in the eyes. The discharges are slight, with the exception of the tears, which are usually profuse and burning, with photophobia (Rhus). The aggravation is usually in the evening, and often concomitant symptoms, such as drowsiness, absence of thirst, etc., are present. This remedy is not frequently called for, though useful when the above indications are present.

Arsenicum. Especially useful when the cornea has become affected and the pustules have broken, leaving *superficial ulceration.* The *photophobia is usually intense* at all times, though it may be so relieved in the open air that the child will open its eyes easily. The lachrymation is profuse, *burning and excoriating, as are all the discharges from the eye*, which are also thin in character. The conjunctival redness is variable; it may be very great, even to chemosis. The pains are generally of a burning character and may be very severe; the eye often feels very hot. The lids may be œdematous and spasmodically closed or else red, inflamed and excoriated by the acrid discharges. The nostrils and upper lip are usually excoriated by the acrid coryza. It is especially indicated in low, cachectic conditions and for the ill-nourished, scrofulous children of the poor. Great restlessness and thirst for small quantities of water are commonly noticed.

Aurum met. Scrofulous ophthalmia with ulceration and vascularity of the cornea. Photophobia severe, lachrymation profuse and scalding; eyes very sensitive to the touch. The pains are from without inward and worse upon touch (reverse of Asafœtida). The cervical glands are usually swollen; patient very irritable and sensitive to noise.

Baryta. Both the carbonate and iodide have been employed in scrofulous ophthalmia, especially when complicated with *enlarged cervical glands*. We have obtained better results from the iodide than from the carbonate.

Belladonna. Rarely useful except in acute aggravations in which there is great photophobia.

Calcarea carb. Particularly indicated in phlyctenular keratitis, though it has also been successfully used in conjunctivitis. Is applicable to this form of inflammation occurring after the suppression of an eruption by mercury, if there is also deafness; also when the disease can be traced to exposure to wet. We usually, though not always, find excessive photophobia and lachrymation (often acrid). The amount of redness is variable, as is also the character of the pain, though this is more commonly described as sticking than otherwise. The lids may be red, swollen and agglutinated in the morning. There is a general *aggravation of the eye-symptoms during damp weather* or from the least cold, to which the patient is very susceptible. It is especially the remedy for pustular inflammation, occurring in *fat*, *unhealthy*, *strumous children* who have enlarged glands, distended abdomen, pale, flabby skin, eruptions on the head and body, which burn and itch, and cold sweat of the head. In fact, upon the concomitant symptoms we place our chief reliance, as the eye symptoms are not characteristic.

Calcarea iod. The indications are nearly the same as for Calcarea carb., though it is preferable in cases in which we have considerable swelling of the tonsils and cervical glands.

Chamomilla. Has proved very serviceable in scrofulous ophthalmia occurring in *cross*, *peevish children during dentition* and will often relieve the severity of the symptoms, even though it does not complete the cure. The cornea is usually invaded and we have great intolerance of light, considerable redness and lachrymation.

Cinnabaris. The cornea is generally implicated in the trouble and the symptoms of photophobia, lachrymation, etc., are severe. *Pain from the inner canthus across the eyebrows* or extending around the eye is a very marked indication for Cinnabaris.

Clematis. Conjunctivitis pust. with tinea capitis over the greater part of the head and agglutination in the morning.

Conium mac. When the inflammation is chiefly confined to the cornea and we have *intense photophobia and profuse lachrymation* upon any attempt to open the spasmodically closed lids. The pains are various, but are generally worse at night. With all this intense photophobia, etc., there is, however, *very slight or no redness of the conjunctiva*, not sufficient to account for the severity of the symptoms.

Croton tig. In both phlyctenular keratitis and conjunctivitis is this drug useful. These are usually complicated by a corresponding characteristic eruption on the face and lids; the eyes and face feel hot and burning, especially at night; the photophobia is marked, ciliary injection like iritis often present, and considerable pain in and around the eye, usually worse at night.

Euphrasia. A valuable remedy in phlyctenular opthalmia when the *lachrymation is excessive*, *acrid* and burning or when there is a *profuse*, *thick*, *acrid*, *muco-purulent discharge which excoriates the lids*, making them red, inflamed and sore; from this discharge the cheek may look as if varnished. Intolerance of light is generally, though not always, present and the conjunctiva may be red even to chemosis. The pains are not marked, though usually of a smarting character from the nature of the discharges. *Blurring of the eyes*, *relieved by winking*, dependent upon the secretions temporarily covering the cornea, especially indicates Euphrasia. Fluent coryza, acrid in character, often accompanies the above symptoms.

Graphites. This is one of the most important remedies we possess for this disease, and its sphere of action is not limited to any special variety, for excellent results have been gained from its use in both the acute and chronic form, whether the cornea is involved or not; it is, perhaps, more often called for in phlyctenular keratitis of the chronic recurrent form. Is especially indicated in scrofulous subjects, covered with eczematous eruptions, chiefly on the head and behind the ears, which eruptions are glutinous, fissured, and bleed easily. The *photophobia is usually intense* and the lachrymation profuse, though, in some cases, nearly or entirely absent; generally worse by daylight than gaslight, and in the morning, so that often the child cannot open the eyes before 9 or 10 A. M. The redness of the eye is generally important (there may be pannus), the discharges muco-purulent, constant, thin and excoriating. The pains are not important and vary; may be sticking, burning, aching or itching. The lids are red, sore and agglutinated in the morning or else covered with dry scales, while the *external canthi are cracked and bleed easily upon opening the eye.* We often notice a *thin, acrid discharge from the nose* accompanying the eye affection.

Hepar sulph. Is most useful in the severer forms of pustular inflammation, especially when upon the cornea and when ulceration has already commenced. The intensity of the symptoms suggests its use such as *intense photophobia*, *lachrymation and great redness of the eye*, *even to chemosis.* The pains are severe, generally of a *throbbing*, stinging character, *ameliorated by warmth*, (so that one wishes to keep the eye covered) and aggravated by cold or uncovering the eye; also usually worse at night or in the evening. The lids are often swollen, spasmodically closed and very sensitive to touch; also may be *red, swollen and bleed easily upon opening.* Particularly indicated in scrofulous, outrageously cross children who have eruptions and boils on various portions of the body.

Kali bichrom. Is adapted to phlyctenules on the conjunctiva or to chronic cases of low grade. The chief characteristics are *absence of photophobia and of redness*, or much less of each than would be expected from the nature of the disease. The pains and lachrymation are also generally absent or nearly so. The eye is often quite sensitive to touch and its secretions are of a stringy character. This form of potash has been more often employed than any other, though the Iodide is also useful in similar cases.

Mercurius. Mercury, in some form, is a frequent remedy for strumous ophthalmia, especially when the cornea has become involved. As the symptoms are similar in all the preparations, we shall at first, under this general head, give those symptoms common to all forms and afterwards give the special indications for each. This is the first remedy to be thought of when this form of inflammation occurs in *syphilitic subjects* whether hereditary or acquired. Especially useful when the cornea is invaded and the vascularity is great, though sometimes there may be a well-marked grayish infiltration around the pustule or ulcer. The redness of the conjunctiva is usually great, even amounting to chemosis, the dread of light is generally great and often intense, so that the patients cannot open their eyes even in a darkened room, and it is more often *aggravated by any artificial light*, as gaslight, the glare of a fire, etc. The *lachrymation is profuse, burning and excoriating*, and the *muco-purulent discharges thin and acrid.* The *pains are generally severe*, varying in character, though more often tearing, burning, shooting or lancinating and are not confined to the eye but extend to the forehead and temples, seeming to lie deep in the bones; they are *always aggravated at night*, especially before midnight, by heat, extreme cold, and in damp weather and are temporarily relieved by cold water. The lids are often spasmodically closed, thick, red, swollen, excoriated from the acrid lachrymation and sensitive to heat or cold and also to contact. The concomitant symptoms of excoriation of the nose, condition of the tongue, eruption on the face, pain in the bones, etc., etc., are of the first importance in selecting this drug.

Mercurius corr. Indicated in the erethistic form of inflammation, occurring in strumous subjects. The pustules are usually found upon the cornea, and hence the severity of the symptoms so marked under this preparation of Mercury, which is more useful than solubilis in severe cases, the pains are more severe, photophobia more marked, lachrymation more profuse and excoriating and all the symptoms more intense than under any preparation we have. Pustules on the cheek, enlarged cervical glands, coated tongue, excoriating coryza, etc., are usually present.

Mercurius dulc. Calomel dusted into the eye has been employed for many years by the old school in scrofulous ophthalmia and even now is considered one of their chief remedies. We also have found this remedy, given internally in the potencies, very useful, in the severer forms of this inflammation, occurring in pale, flabby, scrofulous subjects.

Mercurius nitras. This remedy seems to be particularly adapted to this form of inflammation and has been used, especially by Dr. Liebold, with remarkable success, in a large number of cases. Severe as well as mild, chronic as well as acute cases, superficial as well as deep ulcers have yielded to its influence; in some cases there has been much photophobia, in others none at all, in some severe pain, in others none. We might thus go through a variety of symptoms differing as much as the above, where this drug has proved curative. It is commonly used both externally and internally at the same time, and in the lower potencies, say about the first potency, ten grains to two drachms of water (or even stronger) as an external application, to be used in the eye, two, three or more times a day, and the second, or third potency to be taken internally. Atropine is sometimes used with it, especially when there is considerable photophobia present.

Mercurius præc. rub. This varies little from the general description given of Mercury, it is often used in strumous ophthalmia with great benefit.

Mercurius prot. Not as often required as the other forms of Mercury, unless there be quite extensive superficial ulceration of the cornea, with much photophobia and nocturnal aggravation. There is also usually swelling of the glands, and the *tongue has a thick, yellow coating at the base.*

Mercurius sol. Is very often employed in scrofulous ophthalmia; the indications correspond very closely in all points to those found under the head of Mercurius.

Mezereum. Pustular conjunctivitis, accompanied by eczema of the face and lids, especially when characterized by thick, hard scabs, from under which pus exudes on pressure.

Natrum mur. Especially useful in chronic cases and *after the use of caustics* (*Nitrate of silver*). The eye-symptoms are not particularly characteristic; we have itching, burning and feeling of sand in the eyes, worse in the morning and forenoon; the pains are various though not severe, except perhaps sharp pain over the eye upon looking down, a symptom which we have frequently verified. The lachrymation is acrid and excoriating, making the lids red and sore; the discharges from the eye are also thin, watery and acrid. The photophobia is usually marked, and the lids spasmodically closed. The skin of the face, around the eyes, is often *glossy and shining*, while throbbing headache and other concomitant symptoms are generally present.

Nux vom. Favorable results have been gained in *cases previously much medicated*, both externally and internally. Rarely of service when the conjunctiva only is affected as the most characteristic indications are *excessive photophobia and morning aggravation of all symptoms*, which are indications that the cornea is implicated. The lachrymation is usually profuse and the pains variable, as follows: sharp, darting pains in the eye and over it, in some cases extending to the top of the head and always worse in the morning, burning pains in the eyes and lids; a sense of tearing in the eye at night on awaking from sleep; eye feels pressed out whenever she combs her hair; sensation as of hot water in the eye, pain in the lower lid as if something were cutting it, etc. Sometimes relief from the pain is obtained by bathing the eyes in cold water.

Psorinum. Especially adapted to all *chronic cases of recurrent scrofulous ophthalmia.*

Pulsatilla. This is one of our sheet anchors in the treatment of this disease, especially when the *pustules are confined to the conjunctiva.* It is particularly indicated in persons, especially amenorrhœic females, of a mild temperament and fair complexion, and is also very suitable to this class of ailments when occurring in the negro. When pain in the ear, otorrhœa and other aural symptoms complicate the eye disorder, this remedy would be suggested to our minds. The dread of light is often absent or quite moderate and the redness varies. The lachrymation is not acrid, but more abundant in the open air, while the other *discharges are generally profuse, thick, white or yellow and bland.* The pains vary greatly, but are more often of a pressing, stinging character. The lids may be swollen, though not excoriated, but are very *subject to styes,* for which Pulsatilla is one of our chief remedies. The eyes feel worse on getting warm from exercise or in a heated room and generally in the evening, but are *ameliorated in the open air* and by cold applications. The concomitant symptoms of stomach derangement, amenorrhœa, etc., must be taken into consideration.

Rhus tox. Useful in pustular inflammation after it has progressed to superficial ulceration of the cornea; for then we have present the *intense photophobia and profuse lachrymation* so characteristic of this drug. The conjunctiva may be very red, even to *chemosis, and the lids œdematous, particularly the upper, and spasmodically closed, so that we are compelled to open them by force, when a profuse gush of tears takes place.* The skin of the face, around the eyes, is often covered by a Rhus eruption; especially suitable in a rheumatic diathesis. The symptoms are usually worse at night, after midnight and in damp weather; the patients are restless at night, and disturbed by bad dreams. Rhus rad. has been employed with excellent results in scrofulous ophthalmia when the above symptoms were present. In what respect it differs from Rhus tox., remains to be shown.

Sepia. Especially of value in pustular inflammation found in women, either *occuring with or dependent upon uterine troubles*, and these disorders should receive due consideration in selecting this drug. More often called for when the cornea is affected than when the inflammation is confined to the conjunctiva. The pains are usually of a drawing, aching, piercing character; and aggravated by rubbing, pressing the lids together or pressing upon the eye. The light of day dazzles and causes the head to ache. The conjunctiva may be swollen, with agglutination of the eyes morning and evening, considerable purulent discharge, edges of the lids raw and sore, feeling as if the lids were too tight and did not cover the ball, eruption on the face, etc. *All the symptoms are worse in the morning and evening*, and better in the middle of the day.

Sulphur. This is the remedy, *par excellence*, for pustular inflammation of the cornea or conjunctiva. Its sphere of action is very wide and adapts it to a great variety of cases, especially when *chronic and occurring in scrofulous children covered with eruptions* (and the majority of cases are found in this class), or when otorrhœa and affection of the bones complicate the difficulty; also to those cases which have been caused by suppressing an eruption with external applications. The pains vary, though usually of a *sharp, lancinating character, as if a needle or splinter were piercing the eye*, and may occur at any time of the day or night; or we may have a *sharp shooting pain going through the eye back into the head, from* 1 *to* 3, A. M., which disturbs the sleep of the patients; although, besides these, there may be a variety of other sensations as smarting, itching and burning in the eyes, feeling of pressure as from a foreign body; burning, as from lime; biting as if salt were in the eye; sensations as if there were a number of little burning sparks on the lids, which cause them to close spasmodically; painful dryness as if the lids rubbed the eye ball, bruised pain, etc.. etc. The photophobia is generally very marked and the lachrymation profuse, though in some cases they may be almost or entirely absent. The redness varies greatly, but is usually considerable, especially at the angles; the secretions also vary both in quantity and quality, being often, however, acrid and corroding and sometimes tenacious. Agglutination in the morning is commonly present. The lids are often swollen, burn and smart as if bathed in some acrid fluid, or there is an itching sensation compelling the patient to rub them most of the time. They are frequently covered with an eruption, as well as the surrounding integument of the head and face. All the symptoms are, as a rule, *aggravated by bathing the eyes; so that the child cannot bear to have any water touch them;* also usually worse in the open air.

Tellurium. Has proved successful in phlyctenular conjunctivitis with eczema impetiginoides on the lids and much purulent discharge from the eyes, especially when *complicated with an offensive otorrhœa*, smelling like fish brine.

Zincum. Favorable results have been obtained for the persistent redness of the eye remaining after postular keratitis without any discharge, especially when the redness is more marked at the inner angle and worse toward evening and in the open air.

The following remedies have also proved serviceable in scrofulous ophthalmia, though not so commonly called for as the above: Antimon. tart., Argentum nit., Caust., China, Chloral, Cuprum al., Ferrum, Ferrum iod., Hyoscyamus, Kreosote, Lachesis, Magnet., Magnes. carb., Nitric acid, Petroleum, Phosphorus, Sulphur iod., Thuya.

OPHTHALMIA TRAUMATICA AND ECCHYMOSIS.

The first point to which our attention should be directed, is the removal of any exciting cause, as a foreign body, etc. (See injuries of conjunctiva.)

Applications of cold water or a solution of one of the remedies named hereafter are advised, unless due to some chemical injury.

A compress bandage seems often to hasten the absorption of any hemorrhage into the conjunctiva.

Aconite. There is no remedy more frequently useful than this, in *inflammatory conditions of the eye, resulting from the irritant action of foreign bodies*, as chips of steel, stone or coal, which produce a variable amount of redness and pain, with a sensation of *dryness*, *heat* and burning in the eye.

Arnica. This is probably the most important remedy we possess for *traumatic conjunctivitis or keratitis, following blows and various injuries* of the eye, and is particularly called for *immediately* after the injury, before the inflammatory symptoms have really set in, though is also useful in the later stages. As a remedy for *sub-conjunctival ecchymoses* it is very highly recommended, and many cases, whether resulting spontaneously or from injuries, have come under our notice, in which prompt relief has been obtained from the use of Arnica. The relaxed condition of the blood-vessels and too fluid conditions of the blood, which predisposes to these hemorrhages in whooping-cough, is often successfully met and corrected by this drug.

Calendula. Useful in traumatic inflammation of the conjunctiva or cornea, *following any operation* or resulting from a cut wound of any description.

Cantharis. Ophthalmia traumatica, *caused from any burn*, as from the flame of a candle, explosion of fire works, etc., especially if characterized by much *burning pain* in the eye, usually requires Cantharis.

Hamamelis. Has proved very beneficial in traumatic conjunctivitis and keratitis, consequent upon the burn of a flame or other injuries, in which there has been excoriating pain, great photophobia, constant acrid lachrymation and great vascularity of the conjunctiva. It also seems to hasten the absorption of conjunctival hemorrhages.

Ignatia. Said to have been employed with benefit in traumatic ophthalmia, with violent pains and sensation as if a grain of sand were rolling around beneath the lids.

Ledum pal. Is especially adapted to *ecchymoses of the conjunctiva* of both traumatic and spontaneous origin; in some cases it has seemed to act quicker than Arnica or Hamamelis.

Nux vom. Spontaneous hemorrhage into the conjunctiva, with or without conjunctivitis, has been successfully treated with this remedy, especially if concomitant symptoms point to its use.

Besides these remedies, Euphras., Hepar, Rhus, Sil., Sulph., and others have been successfully employed; in fact any of those remedies mentioned under catarrhal conjunctivitis may prove serviceable, if the indications given are present.

XEROPHTHALMIA.

Treat by the local application of a weak solution of glycerine and water, to which one per cent. of salt should be added; or better still, by the application of artificial serum.

PTERYGIUM.

This disease, considered by the old school as almost proof against medical treatment, frequently yields very readily to the proper homœopathic remedy, though it is true that we too often meet cases which prove very obstinate to treatment, (probably owing to our incomplete knowledge of the materia medica) and in which we are compelled to resort to operative measures. Numerous methods have been advocated, chief among which are excision, ligation and transplantation; for the description of these we would refer to any of the text-books on the subject.

Argentum nit. *Pterygium of a pink color*, especially if there is considerable discharge from the eye, inflammation better in the open air, unendurable in a warm room, and associated with pain at the root of the nose.

Arsenicum. Pterygium if accompanied by dryness of the lids and burning in the eye, or if there is considerable acrid lachrymation, and discharge which excoriates the lids and cheeks; particularly if the general symptoms of restlessness, thirst, etc., are present.

Calcarea carb. Especially indicated in *pterygium, caused from exposure to wet and cold.* (See case in Part I.)

Chimaphila. We have used this drug in many cases when no marked indications were present, with some success, though have also often failed with it. It is, however, valuable in some instances, and should be thought of.

Zincum. Zinc. has been more frequently employed, and has given greater satisfaction than any other remedy, especially in that form of pterygium which extends from the inner canthus (as it usually does), for the majority of the eye symptoms are found at the inner angle, as will be noted by examination of the provings. The lachrymation is usually profuse and photophobia marked, especially by artificial light; pricking pain, *itching and soreness in the inner angle*, worse at night; also itching and heat in the eyes, worse in the cold air and better in a warm room; external canthi cracked. She sees a green halo around the evening light. There may also be present great *pressure across the root of the nose* and supra-orbital region.

The following remedies have also been employed with advantage in the treatment of pterygium, when suggested by constitutional symptoms or certain general characteristic eye indications:—Lach., Nux mos., Psor., Ratan. Spig. and Sulph.

SYMBLEPHARON AND ANCHYLOBLEPHARON.

Both of these are affections which can only be remedied by the use of the knife.

TUMORS OF THE CONJUNCTIVA.

These may be removed in some cases, according to the nature of the tumor, by the proper selection of our drugs based upon constitutional symptoms, though we are often compelled to have recourse to instrumental interference.

For polypi of the conjunctiva, some benefit has been gained from *Calcarea.* Again we find that *Lyco.* has cured one case, though we have also seen it fail.

INJURIES OF THE CONJUNCTIVA.

These may be of a mechanical or chemical nature. If of the former, are usually dependent upon some foreign body which has lodged on the conjunctiva, and the first point to be attended to, will be its removal, which is generally easily affected. After which directions should be given to bathe the eye in cold water or a weak solution of Aconite, Arnica or Calendula. This will usually suffice, though in severe cases it may be advisable to drop a little olive oil into the eye after removing the foreign body.

Chemical injuries, especially from lime, are, unfortunately, of frequent occurrence and very dangerous in their nature on account of the formation of deep sloughs, which have a great tendency to result in symblepharon. If seen early, we should endeavor to remove as much as possible of the lime, and then drop into the eye either a little olive oil, oil of sweet almonds, milk, weak solution of vinegar or some substance which will unite with the lime and form an innocuous compound. Water should never be employed. Great care should be taken while the wound is healing, that no adhesions between the lids and ball occur. If there is a tendency in this direction, the adhesions should be broken up once or twice a day by means of a probe.

When the injury is from some strong acid, as sulphuric or nitric, the eye should be syringed out with a weak solution of carbonate of soda or potassa, in order to neutralize the acid; afterwards olive oil should be dropped in.

CORNEA.

KERATITIS SUPERFICIALIS, KERATITIS ULCEROSA, ULCUS CORNEÆ (CUM HYPOPION), ABSCESSUS CORNEÆ, KERATITIS SUPPURATIVA.

For superficial inflammation of the cornea, very little is required in the way of local treatment, except, perhaps, in severe cases, when a bandage may prove useful. Atropine is employed by the old school in the vast majority of cases, though we, as homœopaths are able to do without it, except in very rare cases with much deep ciliary injection, when it may prove of advantage in connection with remedies.

(*Canthoplasty* has been recommended and performed with benefit in all kinds of inflammation of the cornea, especially in pannus and phlyctenular keratitis, when there is great photophobia and many symptoms of ciliary irritation. It acts chiefly by removing the pressure of the lids from the ball, and should not be made, unless we find that the lid tension is too great.)

In the treatment of ulcers and abscesses of the cornea, local and dietetic measures are of great importance. If the ulcer is extensive, the patient should be directed to remain quiet in the house (in bed, if possible), that absolute rest may be obtained.

As this disease is more often found in weak, debilitated subjects, a very nutritious diet should be prescribed, and it may even be necessary to use stimulants.

As a rule, cold applications are injurious, except, perhaps, in the first or inflammatory stage of the superficial form, though of late ice bags constantly applied to the eye in cases of deep, indolent ulcers on a cornea, covered with pannus and very vascular and soft, have been followed by favorable results.

Upon the other hand, *bandaging* is our most important aid in the treatment, even in some cases producing a cure alone.

In all cases in which the ulcer or abscess is deep, and obstinate to treatment, a protective bandage should be immediately applied. It is usually sufficient to bandage only the affected eye (if one be healthy), unless the ulcer be very deep and extensive, when both eyes should be covered. The objects of the bandage are: to keep the eye quiet and protected by its natural coverings (the lids), to avoid all irritating causes, such as wind, dust, etc., and to keep the eye warm, in order to promote local nutrition.

Atropine is not advised in ulcers or abscesses of the cornea, unless the ulcer is central and has a tendency to perforate, or when iritis complicates the corneal trouble; then atropine should be employed until full dilatation of the pupil is produced, which should be maintained. (A weak solution, one eighth to one grain to the ounce, is usually sufficient to do this.)

External applications are rarely necessary, though we have sometimes seen good results follow the external use of the same drug we are giving internally. (Aqua chlorinata used locally, has also proved beneficial in some cases, especially in the crescentic form and when the discharge of pus is profuse. It may be used pure or diluted one half, one third, or even more.)

In obstinate cases, when the ulcer is extensive and deep, having a great tendency to perforate, "Sæmisch's incision" is recommended. It consists in cutting through the ulcer into the anterior chamber, with a Graefe's cataract knife, which is entered in the healthy tissue on one side, and brought out in the healthy tissue on the other side of the ulceration, which is then divided by a sawing movement of the knife; after which atropine is instilled and a compress bandage applied. The wound can be kept open by the aid of a spatula or Daviel's spoon, for two or three days if desirable.

Paracentesis may also be resorted to in the above cases, though it has been nearly supplanted by "Sæmisch's incision" which, in the majority of instances, is far preferable. All cases of ulcers should be closely watched, that we may detect any hernia of the cornea or prolapse of the iris as soon as it occurs. If a prolapse has taken place, and is of recent origin, we should endeavor to replace it, either by dilating or contracting the pupil, according to its situation, and if this proves inadequate, it should be snipped off with a pair of scissors, atropine instilled and a pressure bandage applied.

Aconite. Superficial ulceration of the cornea of *traumatic origin.* First stage of ulceration caused from exposure in the open air. Conjunctiva very red, even to chemosis, photophobia and lachrymation; or more commonly the eye is *dry*, hot, *burning* and very sensitive to air. Patient restless, feverish, and thirsty.

Apis. Ulceration of the cornea, vascular, with photophobia, hot lachrymation, and burning, *stinging pains;* sometimes the pains are very severe and *shoot* through the eye, with swollen, *œdematous condition of the lids* and conjunctiva. Patient drowsy and thirstless.

Argent. nit. *Ulceration of the cornea in new-born infants, or from any form of purulent ophthalmia, with profuse discharge from the eyes.* Ulceration with halo around the light by day, also with pains like darts through the eye, morning and evening. The pains are usually better in the cool, open air and aggravated in a warm room. The lids are generally red, thick, and swollen, conjunctiva chemosed and the *discharge of whitish yellow pus profuse.*

Arnica. Traumatic ulceration with much *hemorrhage into the anterior chamber.* (Superficial traumatic ulceration generally yields more readily to Acon.)

Arsenicum. Especially when found in scrofulous, anæmic, restless children. The ulceration is chiefly superficial and has a tendency to recur first in one eye, and then in the other. The *photophobia is usually excessive*, and the *lachrymation hot, burning, acrid and profuse.* The pains are *burning, sticking*, twitching in the eyes, and there may be throbbing, pulsating or tearing around the eye, *worse at night.* The *burning pains* predominate and are worse *at night, especially after midnight*, when the child becomes very restless and cross. Bathing in cold water often aggravates, while warm water may relieve. Eyeballs sore to touch. Conjunctiva quite red, even to chemosis. Marked *soreness on the internal surface of the lids*, which are swollen externally, (œdematous) spasmodically closed and often *excoriated by the acrid discharges.*

Asafœtida. Ulceration accompanied by *iritic pains, which extend from within outwards and are relieved by rest and pressure.*

Aurum. Ulceration of the cornea, especially when occurring during the course of *pannus* and scrofulous ophthalmia. Cornea quite vascular, and the patient very irritable and sensitive to noise. Cervical glands often enlarged and inflamed. The *photophobia* is marked, *lachrymation profuse and scalding, and the eyes very sensitive to touch.* The pains extend from without inwards and are worse on touch (reverse of Asaf.).

Calc. carb. Particularly valuable for *corneal ulcerations found in fat, unhealthy children*, with large abdomens, who sweat much, especially about the head, and are very susceptible to cold air; also in deep, sloughing ulcers found in weak cachectic individuals (for which the *hypophosphite* is more commonly employed and often seems to act better than the carb.). The pains, redness, photophobia and lachrymation are variable, and though it is a prominent remedy for this disorder, there are no characteristic eye symptoms, and we are guided in its selection chiefly by concomitant indications. The *iodide of calcarea* is to be preferred in very strumous subjects if accompanying the ulceration, we have *enlargement of the tonsils and cervical glands.*

Cantharis. Superficial ulceration caused by burns, with *burning* pain and lachrymation.

Chamomilla. Ulceration occurring in cross, peevish children during dentition.

China. Ulceration of the cornea of *malarial origin* or dependent upon *anæmic conditions*, especially when the iris has become affected and there are *severe pains*, either in or above the eye, which are *periodic in character*, especially when accompanied by chills. Ulcers found in the course of pannus with much pain in the morning. (For the above symptoms, better results have been obtained from Chin. mur. than from any other preparation.—NORTON.)

Cimicifuga. Ulcers with *sharp, neuralgic pains through the eye into the head.*

Cinnabaris. When accompanied by that characteristic *pain above the eye, extending from the internal to the external canthus, or running around the eye.* This pain varies greatly both in intensity and character. Photophobia and lachrymation are usually present.

Conium. An important remedy in superficial ulceration when the *surface* of the cornea only is abraded; and thus, owing to the exposure of the terminal filaments of the nerve or to hyperæsthesia, there is *intense photophobia* and much lachrymation, so frequently verified clinically under this drug. On account of the great photophobia, the lids are spasmodically closed, and when opened, a profuse gush of tears occurs (Rhus). The discharges are usually slight and the pains variable, though aggravated by any light. But, notwithstanding all this photophobia, pain and lachrymation, we find upon examination, *very little or no redness of the conjunctiva*, not sufficient to account for the great photophobia, which is out of all proportion to the amount of trouble. Strumous conditions, enlarged glands, etc., would assist us.

Croton tig. Ulceration, with marked pain in the supraciliary region at night, especially when accompanied by a *vesicular eruption on the face and lids.*

Euphrasia. Superficial ulceration (sometimes with pannus) may often be relieved, though it rarely affects beneficially any extensive ulceration, except to palliate the symptoms in the first stage.

Photophobia is generally present, as well as *profuse acrid, burning lachrymation*, together with *profuse, acrid, yellowish-white, muco-purulent discharge from the eyes*, which makes the lids red and excoriated, giving them and the cheek an appearance as if varnished.

The conjunctiva is quite red, and the eyes smart and burn. *Blurring of the eyes relieved by winking.*

Graphites. A very valuable remedy in ulceration of the cornea, especially when occurring in scrofulous children who are covered with eczematous eruptions, particularly on the head and *behind the ears;* eruptions are *moist, fissured and glutinous.* Is especially adapted to *superficial ulcerations result-*

ing from pustules, though has also been useful in deep ulcers even with hypopion. The cornea is more frequently found quite vascular and conjunctiva much injected, though both may be slight in degree. The *photophobia is usually intense* and the lachrymation profuse, but may be very moderate in amount. The pains are variable, and the discharges generally thin and excoriating. The lids are sometimes covered with *dry scales*, (the edges) though are more commonly red and sore, with *cracking and bleeding of the external canthi* upon any attempt to open the eyes. Generally accompanying the above symptoms we find an acrid discharge from the nose, which makes the nostrils sore and covered with scabs.

Hamamelis. When dependent upon a blow or burn, especially if complicated with hemorrhage into the anterior chamber (hypæmia).

Hepar. This is one of the best remedies we possess for ulcers and abscesses of the cornea, especially for the *deep, sloughing form, and when hypopion is present.* Some torpid forms of ulcers and abscesses have been benefited, though usually the symptoms are well pronounced when this drug is indicated, as when there is *intense* photophobia, profuse lachrymation, and *great redness of the cornea and conjunctiva*, even to chemosis. The *pains are severe, and of a throbbing*, aching, stinging character, *ameliorated by warmth and aggravated by cold*, or *uncovering the eye* and in the evening.

There is marked *sensitiveness of the eye to touch.* The lids are often red, swollen, spasmodically closed, and *bleed easily upon opening them. For the absorption of pus in the anterior chamber*, (hypopion) *there is no better remedy than Hepar.* Cases found among strumous, outrageously cross children, should suggest this drug. General symptoms of chilliness, etc., are important.

Kali bichrom. Especially of value in those cases of *indolent ulceration* which prove so intractable to treatment, cases in which there is no active inflammatory process, only a low grade of chronic inflammation, therefore marked by *no photophobia and no redness.* The pains are generally slight and variable, and the discharge, if any, of a *stringy character.*

Mercurius sol. Mercury, in some one of its preparations, is a common prescription for ulcers and abscesses; and as the soluble mercury of Hahnemann is perhaps more commonly employed than any other, we shall describe this more definitely, and afterwards give simply the variations of the other forms.

Is adapted to both superficial and deep ulceration, especially when found in a *syphilitic* or strumous subject. The cornea at the point of ulceration is usually quite vascular, though may be surrounded by a grayish opacity, due to infiltration of pus between its layers; the conjunctival redness is also marked. The dread of light is generally great, especially in artificial light, and the lachrymation is profuse, *burning* and *excoriating*, while the discharges are *thin and acrid* in character. The pains are often severe and vary in character, but are *always aggravated at night* by damp weather or extreme cold, and ameliorated temporarily by cold water. The lids are thick, *red*, *swollen and excoriated* by the *acrid discharges*, sensitive to extreme heat or cold, and to contact, and are forcibly closed. The concomitant symptoms of excoriation of the nostrils, flabby tongue, night sweats, pain at night, etc., are usually present.

Mercurius corr. Especially called for when the symptoms found under the previous drug are very marked and severe, particularly if the iris has become complicated with the corneal trouble. The *photophobia*, *acrid lachrymation*, *discharges*, *pains*, *and burning and excoriation of the lids*, are *excessive* (which are more often found in the scrofulous diathesis).

Mercurius dulc. Deep or superficial ulcers or abscesses found in pale, flabby, strumous children, with enlarged glands and general scrofulous cachexia. Other symptoms vary little from Merc. sol., but it is especially valuable in the above subjects.

Mercurius nitr. Has been used empirically with excellent success in all kinds of ulceration, both in the acute and chronic, superficial and deep forms, whether accompanied by hypopion or not, in cases in which there is much photophobia, and in cases in which there is none; where there is much pain, and where there is none. In fact, it has been successfully used in all imaginable forms of the disease, but it seems to act better in those cases in which there is a tendency to the formation of pustules. It is generally employed both externally and internally at the same time, and in the lower potencies; about the first potency in water externally, and the third internally. (Atropine is often used with it, especially when there is much photophobia. Liebold.)

Mercurius præc. rub. Ulceration of a cornea covered with pannus, lids granular, and usual eye symptoms of mercury.

Mercurius prot. *Serpiginous ulceration* of the cornea, that commences at the margin and *extends over the whole cornea, or a portion of it, especially the upper part, involving only the superficial layers.* This form of ulceration is more commonly found during the course of *trachoma and pannus*, and the protoïodide of Mercury has often proved its value in these cases.

The *vascularity of the cornea and conjunctiva* is great, while the *photophobia is usually excessive.* The pains are the same as those given under Mercurius sol. A *thick yellow coating at the base of the tongue* is generally present.

Natrum mur. Ulcers that appear *after the use of caustics*, particularly the nitrate of silver. Photophobia usually marked, so that a child will lie with the head buried in the pillows, *lachrymation acrid*, discharges thin and excoriating, lids swollen, eruption around the eye on face, which is often *shining*, pains various, though often *sharp and piercing above the eye on looking down*, are the most prominent eye indications. Concomitants will decide our choice.

Nux vom. *Superficial ulceration* of the cornea, characterized by *excessive photophobia, especially in the morning;* during the day is often comparatively free from it. The amount of redness is not usually excessive, though varies, as does also the character of the pains. Lachrymation is profuse. To be thought of in cases that have been previously overdosed with medicine, both externally and internally. Neuro-paralytic inflammation of the cornea has been benefited.

Pulsatilla. Superficial ulcers following phlyctenules, occurring in females of a mild temperament. *Thick, bland*, white or yellow discharge from the eyes, and general *amelioration of symptoms in the open air.* (Not a common remedy.)

Rhus tox. *Superficial keratitis with excessive photophobia and lachrymation, so that the tears gush out upon opening the spasmodically closed lids;* if a child, will often lie with its face buried in the pillows all day. *Profuse flow of tears* is a very important symptom under this drug, and benefit is frequently derived from its use in *superficial ulceration of the cornea with granular lids* in which this symptom is often prominent. Keratitis caused from *exposure to the wet*, often calls for Rhus. (Calc.)

The redness of the eye is generally marked, even to *chemosis of the conjunctiva. The lids are œdematously swollen, especially the upper.* An eruption may frequently be found around the eye, characteristic of the drug.

The symptoms are *generally worse in damp weather and at night after midnight*, therefore the patients are restless at night and disturbed by bad dreams. A rheumatic diathesis would also influence our choice.

Secale. Suppuration of the cornea *aggravated by warm applications*, has been cured.

Silicea. Adapted to *sloughing ulcers* of the cornea, and also to *small round ulcers* which have a tendency to perforate, especially if situated near the centre of the cornea and having no blood-vessels running to them. Pain, photophobia, lachrymation, redness and discharges vary, though the latter is generally profuse in the sloughing form of the disease. Hypopion may be present. The silicea patient is usually *very sensitive to cold* and therefore wishes to keep wrapped up warm, especially about the head.

Sulphur. Beneficial results have followed the use of this drug in all varieties of ulcers and abscesses, from the simple abrasion of the epithelial layer following the disappearance of a phlyctenule, to the most severe sloughing form of ulcers or abscesses we may see. Both acute and chronic cases have been relieved, though it is more often to be thought of in the latter form, even in cases in which the destruction of tissue is great and *pus is present in the anterior chamber*, especially if the inflammation be indolent in nature, with no photophobia and slight vascularity.

Ulcerations occurring in, or dependent upon a *scrofulous diathesis*, as shown by eruptions etc., very quickly suggest this remedy, as does also any case which can be traced to the suppression of an eruption. The most prominent eye indications which would lead us to the selection of this drug, are the pains, which are usually *sharp and sticking, as if a needle or splinter were sticking in the eye*, or there may be *sharp, shooting pains through the eye into the head from one to three A. M.* (These severe pains through the eye into the head, during the day or evening, rarely call for Sulphur, but for Spig., Bry., Cimicif., or the like); again we may have a great variety of other sensations (See Sulphur) Part I. The *intolerance of light is generally great* and the *lachrymation profuse*, though both are variable. All the symptoms are, as a rule, *aggravated by bathing the eyes*, so that a child cannot bear to have any water touch them.

Thuya. Ulcerations of a syphilitic origin, even when hypopion is present, suffusion of the eyes and burning in them. Pain over them as if a nail were being driven in, etc.

Vaccinium. Ulcers appearing after vaccination.

The following remedies have also been followed by favorable results in occasional cases:—Alumina, Baryta carb. and jod., Bell., Caust., Chin. ars., Kali carb. and jod., Kreos., Nit. ac., Sang., Seneg. and Sepia.

KERATITIS PHLYCTENULARIS.

(See conjunctivitis phlyctenularis.)

KERATITIS PANNOSA (PANNUS).

For treatment, both local and constitutional, see *conjunctivitis trachomatosa;* also compare remedies under *keratitis superficialis* for special indications.

The following are, however, most frequently called for:—

Arg. nit., Ars., *Aurum*, Cannab., *Chin. mur.*, *Graph.*, *Hepar*, Kali carb., Merc. sol., *prot.* and *præc. rub.*, Nat. mur., *Petrol.*, Puls., Rhus, *Sulph.*

KERATITIS TRAUMATICA.

(See ophthalmia traumatica.)

KERATITIS PARENCHYMATOSA.

In the treatment of this, the interstitial variety of inflammation of the cornea, our main dependence is placed upon constitutional treatment with our remedies; and here homœopathy shows its great advantage over the old school, for we can often check the progress of the disease in a speedy manner, by the careful selection of our drugs.

As the general health of our patients is not usually very good, plenty of exercise in the open air and a nutritious diet, are to be especially advised.

No external applications should be made, except in rare cases in which the ciliary injection is great and there seems to be iritic complication, when atropine can be employed with benefit.

Paracentesis and an iridectomy are to be thought of as a last resort, or when there is increase of the intra-ocular tension.

Aurum mur. This is the preparation of gold we have most commonly used, and in the lower potencies. It is especially important in all those cases in which the cause can be traced to *hereditary syphilis*, and as the majority of cases of genuine interstitial keratitis are of this origin, it can readily be seen how common a remedy this may be. We have seen it act speedily and permanently in both the vascular and non-vascular variety of the disease, though in nearly all cases marked symptoms of an hereditary taint have been present, as shown by the character of the teeth, described by Hutchinson, as well as by the history of the case. The subjective symptoms are not prominent and may be absent, though usually there is some photophobia, irritable condition of the eye, and dull pain in and around the eye, which often seems deep in the bone.

Baryta jod. Interstitial keratitis occurring in scrofulous subjects, *with great enlargement of the cervical glands*, which are hard and painful on pressure.

Hepar. Especially of service in clearing the cornea after the inflammatory process has been checked.

Merc. sol. Some preparation of mercury is often required, as we would be led to expect from its usual specific origin. We would class this remedy with Aurum, as the two most commonly called for. There is generally more redness, pain and iritic complication when mercury is indicated, than we find under Aurum. The *nocturnal aggravation* is also quite marked, as well as the concomitant symptoms.

Sepia. Keratitis parenchymatosa complicated with uterine disturbances.

Sulphur. Indicated in strumous subjects, even when the inflammation is in an active stage. Especially useful, however, in promoting the absorption of the infiltration into the cornea, after the inflammation has been allayed by the proper remedies.

Apis., *Ars.*, Calc. carb., and jod., Cannab. sat., and the Mercurials are also to be kept in mind, as favorable results have been obtained from their use.

KERATO IRITIS.

(Refer to *Iritis* and *Keratitis.*)

LEUCOMA, MACULA, ETC.

Opacities of the cornea usually prove very obstinate to treatment, though many remedies have been recommended and used, to effect their removal.

The old school rely chiefly upon the use of irritants, as

calomel, red and yellow oxide of mercury, etc., to promote absorption; we have also seen good results from irritating substances applied to the opacity, as Cuprum al. and other remedies which are employed at the same time internally, though do not advise them in the majority of cases.

Electricity has been advised for their dispersion.

In order to cut off the irregularly refracted rays of light in some forms of opacities, Stenopaic spectacles either with or without convex or concave glasses, may be of advantage.

An iridectomy opposite a transparent portion of the cornea, is frequently advisable, especially where the opacity is too dense to be removed by remedies.

As there is usually a total lack of eye symptoms in these cases, we must chiefly rely upon the general condition of the patient, though below are to be found those drugs which are more commonly indicated and those which are said to have produced cures. Apis, Aur., Calc., Cannab., *Chel., Crotal., *Cupr. al., Euph., Hepar.,* Kali bichrom., *Nat. sul., Nit. ac., Rhus, Sacch. alb., Sil., Spong., and Sulph.

STAPHYLOMA CORNEÆ.

(*Kerato-conus, Buphthalmus, etc.*)

We have seen the progress of conical cornea checked by the employment of the proper homœopathic remedy, though we believe it is impossible to diminish the conicity of the cornea without instrumental interference. The remedy must be chosen according to both local and constitutional symptoms, though *Calc. jod.* has proved most serviceable in our hands. Suitable hygienic measures are of great importance, as this affection may be dependent upon a debilitated condition of the health. A pressure bandage may sometimes be used with advantage, but if the disease seems still to increase in spite of medication, an

*) These remedies have been usually employed externally, at the same time they were given internally.

iridectomy is required. Either stenopaic or concave glasses may improve the vision.

Various operations are recommended for the cure of conical cornea, as cauterization or removal of a piece from the apex, etc.

Staphyloma of the cornea may be total or partial and either accompanied by protrusion of the iris or not, but our first aim should be, in the treatment of ulcers and other diseases of the cornea which tend toward this sad result, to endeavor to prevent it by bandaging and proper medicinal means. If however, staphyloma is already present, we must have recourse to the knife, and here we find many operations advisable according to the duration and extent of the staphylomatous bulging.

Apis, Ilex aqui fol., and Euphras. are said to have cured staphyloma (!).

XEROSIS CORNEÆ.

(See Xerophthalmia.)

INJURIES AND WOUNDS OF THE CORNEA.

Foreign bodies in the cornea are of frequent occurrence and can usually be easily removed by the aid of a spud without fixing the eye, though if the patient be very nervous and the foreign body imbedded in the cornea, it is better to use a stop speculum and then fix the eye with a pair of forceps. An anæsthetic may be necessary in rare cases. If the foreign body has penetrated the cornea and lies partly in the anterior chamber, a broad needle should be introduced behind it, thus preventing its being pushed backward in our attempt to extract it. Chemical injuries have already been treated of under the conjunctiva.

The treatment of wounds of the cornea varies according to the complications which may arise. We usually, though, endeavor in the first stage to subdue inflammatory symptoms by cold compresses of *Aconite*, *Arnica*, *Calendula* or *Hamamelis*, besides using atropine in the eye; unless the cornea is perforated near the periphery, when better results are to be obtained from Calabar bean. Perfect rest should be insisted upon if the injury be extensive; and if iritis should set in, the cold compresses must be changed to warm.

TUMORS OF THE CORNEA.

(See Conjunctiva.)

SCLERA.

SCLERITIS, EPISCLERITIS AND SCLERO-CHOROIDITIS ANT.

The local symptoms of this disease being usually few and indefinite, we are obliged to derive our indications for remedies from the general symptoms of the patient.

If there is great ciliary injection and pain, a solution of atropine may be employed, but is rarely necessary.

Aconite. In the acute stage, if there are violent, aching, dragging, tearing pains in the eyeballs, with contracted pupils, photophobia, and the characteristic reddish blue circle around the cornea. The eye is usually quite sensitive to touch, and feels hot and dry. Especially useful if caused from cold, or exposure to dry, cold air.

Kalmia. Sclero-choroiditis ant. Sclera inflamed, vitreous filled with opacities, glimmering of light below one eye, especially on reading with the other, were indications present in one case, in which Kalmia was of great service.

Mercurius. Inflammation of the sclerotic, which is thinned so that the choroid shines through. *Steady, aching pain in the eye all the time, but worse at night;* also usually some pain around the eye, especially if the iris has become involved. Particularly to be thought of, if of syphilitic origin. Concomitant symptoms of flabby tougue, offensive breath, night pains, etc., are of great importance.

Silicea. Sclerotic inflamed, with or without choroideal complication. The pains may be severe, and extend from the eyes to the head, and are *relieved by warmth.* Aching in the occiput corresponding to the eye affected.

Thuya. This is a very valuable remedy in all forms of inflammation of the sclera, even if no characteristic symptoms are present. It should be the first remedy suggested to our minds in the treatment of scleritis, sclero-choroiditis, or any of its complications, as clinical experience has often verified its usefulness in these cases. We are unable to give positive indications for its use, but have frequently observed that inflammation and softening of the sclera, resulting from the extension of the inflammation of parenchymatous keratitis, kerato-iritis, and keratitis punctata, have been promptly and uniformly checked by Thuya. In most of these cases there has been great tenderness of the globe, intolerance of light, and active inflammation, with a general cachectic condition, occurring in persons badly nourished, either scrofulous or syphilitic, and those long time deprived of fresh air.

The following have also been used and are recommended: Cocc., *Puls.*, Spig., and Sulph.

STAPHYLOMA SCLERÆ.

We should endeavor to prevent this result by the use of those remedies given under scleritis, but if it seems to progress in spite of our remedies, an *iridectomy* must be made.

If the staphyloma has existed for some time, it will be necessary to abscise it, according to some of the methods advised; or, if it be extensive, and sight is lost, enucleation is to be preferred.

WOUNDS AND INJURIES OF THE SCLERA.

The treatment of wounds of the sclerotic varies according to their extent and situation. If any protrusion of the contents of the globe has occurred, this should be cut off, and the edges of the wound approximated as closely as possible by the aid of a bandage, or the introduction of a fine suture. The patient should be kept quiet in bed, and cold applications of Arnica or Calendula solutions employed, as may be most applicable from the nature of the injury, whether contused or incised.

If the wound, however, is extensive, especially if in the ciliary region, enucleation is far the safer method of proceeding, even though the vision is not wholly lost, in order that all danger of sympathetic trouble in the other (healthy) eye may be taken away. In all cases in which a large portion of the contents of the globe has escaped and sight is irretrievably lost, enucleation is necessary.

If there is a foreign body in the sclerotic it should be removed, but if it has penetrated the sclerotic and is within the eye, it is wiser to enucleate than to attempt its extraction, as a general rule.

IRIS.

IRITIS.

(*Idiopathic, traumatic, syphilitic and serous.*)

The first point that demands our attention is the removal of any cause that remains exciting as for instance, a foreign body in the conjunctiva, cornea or interior of the eye. If it be due to swelling or dislocation of the lens forward, or to a portion of the lens substance lying against the iris, an incision should be made and the irritating object removed. When dependent upon sympathetic irritation from the other eye, which has been already destroyed, enucleation should be performed as early as possible. If previous synechiæ are the exciting causes, an iredectomy becomes necessary.

We are sometimes compelled to treat quite severe cases of this disease as out patients and often with excellent results, though it is far better and safer in all cases to confine the patient to the house. If the patient is allowed to leave the house, the eyes must be carefully guarded by bandaging the affected eye and protecting the other by a shade or colored glass. We should, however, in all cases, especially if severe, most positively insist upon the patient remaining in a darkened room and in bed, in order that perfect rest may be obtained, both from the irritation of light and from muscular movements. A low or milk diet usually proves most beneficial, unless the patient be too much debilitated.

Cold applications should never be employed in iritis, except possibly in the first stage of the traumatic form, when a solution of Arnica or Calendula may be useful, though even then we should prefer warm applications. *Warmth* is one of our most important aids in the treatment and it may be employed in any way, though we especially advise *dry warmth*, covering the eye and corresponding side of the head with lint, hot salt bags, or what is better fine cotton, for by this the heat may be kept more uniform than by the application of moisture.

The next point in the treatment of iritis is one of great importance and should always be attended to, viz.: complete dilatation of the pupil as early as possible by the use of *atropine.* (See atropine, Part I.). As soon as the nature of the disease has been detected, a solution of atropine should be instilled strong enough to produce the desired result, and when the dilatation is complete, we should endeavor to keep it so by a continued application of the mydriatic. If, however, the pupil is already bound down by adhesions which cannot be readily torn, it is better to discontinue the atropine until the inflammatory symptoms have subsided, when it may again be tried to break up the adhesions. A solution of atropine, four grains to the ounce of water, is commonly employed, though it is better to use a weaker solution, even one eighth of a grain to the ounce, if the required effect can be accomplished with this, *but the pupil must be dilated*, if possible, even if we have to employ the crude substance. These remarks regarding atropine will apply to the various forms of iritis, with the exception of the serous variety, in which dilatation is not necessary.

An iridectomy may be made in the later stages, and when other treatment fails; it is also indicated in serous iritis, if glaucomatous symptoms supervene.

Aconite. "In the *very first stage*, or in a sudden re-appearance, this remedy is often of the greatest value," especially if occurring in young, full blooded patients, and when the cause can be traced to an *exposure to a cold draught of air.* The ciliary injection is usually marked, pupils contracted, and pains often severe, beating and throbbing, especially at night. We also have a sensation of *great heat* and dryness in the eyes; symptoms generally accompanied by general febrile excitement.

Arnica. Rheumatic iritis has been benefited, though its special sphere of action is in the *traumatic variety*, in which it is often employed with advantage.

Arsenicum. Iritis with *periodic burning pains*, worse at night, after midnight, ameliorated by warm applications. Frequently indicated in serous iritis.

Asafœtida. *Especially indicated in the syphilitic variety, and after the abuse of mercury.* (More applicable to the female sex. Liebold.) The *pains are severe* in the eye, *above it*, and in the temples, of a *throbbing, pulsating*, pressing, *burning*, or sticking character, and tend to become periodic; they extend usually from *within outwards*, and are *relieved by rest and pressure* (reverse of Aurum).

Aurum. Chiefly serviceable in *syphilitic iritis*, and after overdosing with mercury or potash; when characterized by much *pain which seems to be deep in the bones* surrounding the eye, of a tearing, pressing nature, often extending down into the eyeball, with burning heat, especially on trying to open the eyes; the pressing pain is usually from *above downwards*, and from *without inwards*, aggravated on touch. The vision is clouded as by a dark veil. The mental condition of the patient is that of great depression; this, together with the bone pains in other portions, aids us materially in our choice.

Belladonna. Early stages of iritis, caused from a cold, with much redness and *throbbing pain* in the eye and head, congestion of the face, etc. Is not frequently indicated in iritis.

Bryonia. Iritis resulting from exposure to cold, not unfrequently calls for this drug, especially if occurring in a rheumatic diathesis. The pains may be sharp and *shooting* in the eyes, *extending through into the head*, or *down into the face*, or there may be a sensation of *soreness and aching* in and around the ball, especially behind it, extending through to occiput; the patient also sometimes describes the pain, as *if the eye was being forced out of the socket.* All the pains are generally *aggravated by moving the eyes in their socket, or upon any exertion of them, and at night.* The seat of pain often becomes sore to touch. In the serous form it should also prove serviceable.

Calendula. Traumatic iritis.

Cedron. This remedy is particularly of value in relieving the severe *ciliary neuralgia* observed in iritis, especially if *supra-orbital*, seeming to follow the course of the supra-orbital nerve, especially when there is marked periodicity. In relieving the pain it acts favorably upon the disease by removing nervous irritation, and following the more beneficial action of the true remedy.

China. Iritis dependent upon the *loss of vital fluids*, or malaria. The pains are variable but have a marked *periodicity.* (The Muriate of Quinine in appreciable doses will often relieve the *severity of the pains*, especially when of an *intermittent type and accompanied by chills and fever.* Liebold.)

Cinnabaris, as one of the preparations of mercury, stands high in the treatment of iritis, particularly syphilitic, and when condylomata are present on the iris and even on the lids. The characteristic *pain commences at the inner canthus and extends across the brow, or even passes around the eye,* though there may be shooting pains through the eye into the head, especially at inner canthus, or soreness along the course of the supra-orbital nerve and corresponding side of the head. Like Mercury, the *nocturnal aggravation* is usually marked, and the symptoms intermit in severity.

Clematis. By some this drug is considered to be as frequently called for as Mercury, in iritis and kerato-iritis, though we have never used it to the same extent. The pains are similar to those of Mercurius, but there is usually much heat and dryness in the eye, and great *sensitiveness to cold air*, to light, and bathing. (Is said to have a marked action on the adhesions which take place between the iris and lens.)

Conium. Keratitis punctata with *excessive photophobia*, and but little redness or apparent inflammation.

Euphrasia. Rheumatic iritis with constant aching and occasional darting pain in the eye, always worse at night; ciliary injection and photophobia great, aqueous cloudy, and iris discolored and bound down by adhesions.

Gelsemium. Serous iritis alone or complicated with choroideal exudation, should especially suggest this remedy.

Hamamelis. Iritis traumatica or other forms in which *hemorrhage has taken place into the anterior chamber.*

Hepar. Especially serviceable if the inflammation has extended to the neighboring tissues, corneal ulceration (kerato-iritis), when the ciliary body has become involved, or after condylomata have ruptured, and there is *pus in the anterior chamber* (*Hypopion*). As hypopion is an important symptom under Hepar, we should think of this remedy in parenchymatous or suppurative inflammation of the iris, in which this condition is present. The pains are pressing, boring, or *throbbing*, in the eye, *ameliorated by warmth* and aggravated by motion; *eye often very tender to touch.* There is usually much photophobia and great redness of the conjunctiva, even amounting to chemosis, while the lids may be red, swollen, spasmodically closed, and sore to touch. The patient feels chilly, and wants to keep warmly covered. Payr says that it is the chief remedy for keratitis punctata.

Kali iod. An important remedy in *syphilitic iritis*, especially after mercurialization, and when the secondary eruption on the skin is present. The special indications are not marked, as it has been given upon general principles in many instances, with excellent success.

The bichromate of potash has also been employed in similar cases.

Mercurius. Mercury and its various combinations are our "sheet anchors" in the treatment of *all forms of iritis*, *especially the syphilitic*; and the cases which call for its use present a great variety of symptoms, differing much, both in character and intensity. The *pains are usually severe*, and of a tearing, boring, cutting, burning nature, chiefly around the eyes, and in the forehead and temples, also accompanied by throbbing, shooting and sticking pains in the eye, though in rare cases they may be almost or entirely absent; these pains as well as all the symptoms of the mercurials are *always worse at night*, *after going to bed*, *and in damp weather*, in this respect corresponding very closely to the disease. There is generally much heat both in and around the eye, and soreness of the corresponding side of the head to touch. *Great sensitiveness* to heat or *cold* may be found, *also to light*, *especially the glare of a fire.* Lachrymation (acrid) is often present. The *pupil is contracted*, and *overspread by a thin bluish film*, *while there is great tendency to the formation of adhesions to the lens* (posterior synechiæ). The iris is discolored, aqueous cloudy, and ciliary injection marked. *Hypopion* may be present or not. *Condylomata* may also be found on the iris. The lids may be red, swollen and spasmodically closed, or even normal in appearance. The concomitant symptoms of *nocturnal pains* in different portions of the body, perspiration at night, condition of tongue, mouth, and throat, eruptions on the skin, etc., are of great importance in selecting this drug, and in choosing between the different preparations.

The *Corrosivus* is most frequently employed, and proves most beneficial, as the *intensity* of the symptoms is more marked under this than any other form.

The *Solubis* comes next in order of usefulness, and should be given if the above symptoms are present, and if the inflammation is of medium intensity or lower grade, and if certain characteristic general symptoms are observed.

The *Dulcis* is to be thought of when iritis is found in very scrofulous subjects, especially children, with pale, flabby skin, and when associated with corneal ulceration.

The *Protoiodide* should be chosen from concomitant symptoms, as *thick, yellow coating at the base of the tongue*, enlarged glands, etc., and when superficial ulceration of the cornea complicates the difficulty, especially if found during the course of pannus.

Nitric acid. Especially indicated after suppressed *syphilis*, or the abuse of mercury; also in gonorrhœal kerato-iritis. The pains are usually pressing or stinging, and aggravated on any change of temperature, at night, and on touching the parts. (See Nitric acid.)

Nux vom. May be useful at the beginning of the disease, or as an intercurrent, especially in the syphilitic form, if there is much photophobia, lachrymation, etc., *in the morning*.

Petroleum. Particularly syphilitic iritis, and when accompanied by *occipital headache*. Pain in eyes, pressing or stitching, and skin around the eyes dry and scurfy.

Rhus tox. Idiopathic or rheumatic iritis, especially if the cause can be traced to *exposure to wet* and if found in a rheumatic patient. *Suppurative iritis, particularly if of traumatic origin, as after cataract extraction*, more often calls for Rhus than any other remedy. Also useful in kerato-iritis. *The lids are œdematously swollen, spasmodically closed, and upon opening them a profuse gush of tears takes place. The conjunctiva is also chemosed,* the photophobia marked and the pains various, both in and around the eye, *worse at night,* especially after midnight and in damp weather. The swelling of the lids often involves the corresponding side of the face and may be covered by a vesicular eruption. Concomitants must be taken into consideration.

Silicea. Iritis with hypopion would suggest this remedy if other indicative symptoms are present.

Spigelia. Rheumatic iritis, if the pains are *sharp and shooting, both in and around the eye, especially if they seem to radiate from one point.*

Sulphur. Iritis, particularly when chronic and found in strumous subjects, especially after suppression of eruptions or discharges, may find its remedy in Sulphur; also when *hypopion* complicates the trouble. May often be of service as an intercurrent, even if it does not complete the cure. The pains are usually of a *sharp, sticking character,* worse at night and towards morning. General indications will decide our choice.

Terebinth. Excellent results have been obtained from its employment in iritis, especially of the rheumatic type, if urinary symptoms and suppressed perspiration of the feet have given the indications.

Thuya. *Syphilitic iritis, marked by condylomata on the iris. Large wart-like excrescences on the iris, with severe, sharp, sticking pains in the eye, aggravated at night and ameliorated by warmth.* Usually accompanying the above, we find *much heat* above and around the eye and in the corresponding side of the head; there may also be tearing, dull, aching pains in brow, or a pain above the eye (left), as if a nail were being driven in. *Ciliary injection,* decided even in some cases amounting to inflammation of the sclera. Lids may be indurated, noises in the head, etc.

The following remedies have also been employed in occasional cases with favorable results. Their meagre indications can be found by reference to drugs in Part I. Arg. nit., Cocc., Crot. tig., Hyos., Ledum, Nat. mur., Plumb., Puls., Stilling. and Zinc.

IRIDO-CYCLITIS, IRIDO-CHOROIDITIS AC., CHRON. AND SYPH. OPHTHALMIA SYMPATHICA.

Sympathetic ophthalmia is found in this section, as it usually shows itself in the form of irido-cyclitis, and therefore demands similar treatment.

The first point in the treatment of inflammation of the uveal tract is, to remove any cause that may be present, as can be found under the section of iritis; or, if it be due to sympathetic irritation from the other diseased eye, as is frequently the case, our first indication should always be, to remove the bad eye, even after the prodroma have set in, except in cases in which the inflammatory symptoms are very severe, when it is better to wait until these have subsided in some degree, before the enucleation is performed.

During an acute attack the patient should be confined to the house, in a dark room and in bed with the eye bandaged.

Atropine must be employed as early as possible to break up any iritic adhesions, but if they prove too strong for this drug to tear, we then find an iridectomy advisable.

In old cases, in which the lens has become cataractous, various operations for the removal of the lens have been employed.

Our chief reliance must be placed upon internal medication, and for special indications of each drug we would refer to the therapeutics of iritis and choroiditis. The following remedies however have been more commonly used with advantage, and would be among the first suggested to our minds: Apis, Ars., Asaf., Aur., *Bell.*, *Bry.*, *Kali iod.*, *Merc. corr. and iod.*, Prunus spin., *Rhus*, *Sil.* and Thuya.

SYNECHIÆ, ANTERIOR AND POSTERIOR.

The common results of inflammation of the iris, after improper treatment or no treatment at all, are adhesions of this tissue to the lens or cornea (the latter more often results from ulceration and perforation of the cornea). This condition we are frequently called upon to treat, not only on account of its impairment of vision, but also to remove the cause of constant recurring iritis and other more serious disorders.

The first and most important measure is, to endeavor to tear the adhesions by the use of strong solutions of *atropine* or Calabar bean, or both alternately, according to extent and situation. If we do not succeed by these means, a hook may be introduced and the adhesions torn, though this is a very delicate procedure and is rarely undertaken.

If the ocular tension increases or a chronic inflammation is set up, an iridectomy becomes necessary.

Electricity has been advised and used to promote absorption.

Some remedies, as Clematis, Graph., Merc. corr., Sulph., and Terebinth., seem to have a favorable action upon these adhesions, causing them to absorb or soften so that they can be easily torn by atropine.

MYDRIASIS.

Dilatation of the pupil is usually merely a symptom of some deeper and more serious trouble and therefore requires remedies adapted to that condition. It is sometimes found uncomplicated by any other disorder, though, being dependent upon cold, trauma, etc., in which case Bell., Arnica and a score of remedies may be indicated. (The external application of Calabar bean is also often of great service.) As mydriasis is generally associated with paralysis of some one of the ocular muscles, we would refer for treatment to paralysis of the muscles.

MYOSIS.

Contraction of the pupil unassociated with some more serious disturbance is of rare occurrence; it therefore usually demands treatment for the cause. Atropine instilled into the eye may be employed, though generally gives only temporary relief.

Physostigma ven. is especially recommended for this condition, though various remedies which produce contraction of the pupils may be thought of.

TUMORS OF THE IRIS.

Tumors of the iris are usually more successfully treated by surgical interference, than by internal or external medication.

WOUNDS OF THE IRIS.

If a foreign body be seen lying upon or in the iris, it should be removed by making an iridectomy, excising that portion of the iris, in which the foreign body is situated; after which atropine should be instilled, a bandage applied and the patient put to bed.

When a portion of the iris protrudes through an opening in the cornea, an attempt should be made to replace it by the use of atropine or Calabar bean; if these means fail, it may be excised and the patient treated as after an iridectomy.

Injuries of the iris usually produce iritis, for treatment of which refer to iritis.

Hemorrhage often takes place into the anterior chamber from an injury to the iris, and to hasten the absorption of which a solution of *Arnica* or *Hamamelis* applied externally, usually proves very beneficial. (One case of hemorrhage into the anterior chamber following an iridectomy, in which the blood remained some three weeks without undergoing any apparent absorption, notwithstanding the use of both Arnica and Hamamelis, was absorbed within three days under the use of Ledum, externally and internally.)

CHOROID.

HYPERÆMIA OF THE CHOROID. CHOROIDITIS SEROSA AND DISSEMINATA.

In the treatment of inflammation of the choroid, some have of late advised the confinement of the patient in a dark room and reclining most of the time. This does very well in the acute serous variety, in which we have also seen good results from the use of a bandage at the same time, but in chronic cases and in the disseminate form, we would advise the patient to take moderate exercise in the open air, having the eyes protected from the bright light by blue glasses. The regular instillation of atropine is of great service in many cases, as it paralyzes the tensor choroidea, thus preventing any movement of the inflamed tissue upon every change of light. Complete rest of the eyes from all work should always be required. In the serous variety if the tension becomes increased, an iridectomy is indicated. Abstinence from all stimulants and proper hygienic measures should be attended to.

Aurum. Cases following overdosing by potash or mercury. Choroiditis even when complicated with retinitis, especially if there is a *serous exudation between the choroid and retina*, or into the vitreous, causing haziness of the vitreous. We may have sensitiveness to light and touch, ciliary injection and some pressive pain in the eye, from above downward or from without inward, aggravated on touch, or pain in the bones around the eye. A general feeling of malaise and depression of spirits is usually present.

Belladonna. This is one of our most important drugs for *hyperœmia* or acute inflammatory conditions of the choroid, particularly of the disseminate variety and when accompanied by congested headaches. The optic disk is of a deep red color, and the retinal vessels enlarged, especially the veins. Pupil slightly dilated, ciliary injection usually marked, eyes generally sensitive to light and feel full, as if pressed out of the head. Disturbances of vision are also often present, as halo around the light, various flashes of light, sparks, etc. The headache and constitutional symptoms decide our choice.

Bryonia. *Serous choroiditis* or inflammation of the uveal tract following rheumatic iritis, will often be benefited by this drug. From *serous* infiltration into the vitreous, the haziness is often so great as to seriously interfere with our view of the fundus. The vessels of the fundus are congested; the pupils may be somewhat dilated and the tension increased. *The eyeball feels sore to touch and motion*, while *darting pains through the eye into the head* are often present.

Gelsemium. An important remedy in *serous choroiditis*, especially if the inflammation is situated anterior to the equator, and the serous exudation into the vitreous is great, giving a fine diffused haziness to this humor. The optic nerve will be found hyperæmic and sometimes the retina also, when the fundus can be seen. The tension may be increased and pupils dilated. We may also find some iritic complication and thus a tendency to the formation of adhesions to the lens, accompanied by slight contraction of the pupil. There is a feeling of soreness in the eyeball to touch (Bry.). The vision may vary greatly from day to day or even from hour to hour. In one case small transparent points very sensitive to touch, made their appearance on the surface of the cornea, but disappeared quickly after the use of Gels. Fever sometimes accompanies this condition, though thirstlessness is prominent. The character of the headache is also often a valuable concomitant.

Kali iod. The iodide of potash is very serviceable in inflammation of the choroid, particularly of the *disseminate variety*, especially if traceable to a syphilitic origin, though we have derived great benefit from its employment when no specific history could be obtained, as can be seen by reference to case under Kali iod. Its results are often wonderful, even when atrophic changes in the choroid are far advanced or when the whole uveal tract is involved.

Mercurius. Mercury in some one of its forms (chiefly the corrosivus or solubis), has frequently proved useful in choroiditis, especially of the disseminate form or when the *iris is also involved* (irido-choroiditis). Cases occurring in or dependent upon a *syphilitic dyscrasia*, not rarely demand the employment of mercury, and even cases of a non-syphilitic origin are often decidedly benefited by its use. The tendency to the formation of adhesions between the iris and lens, should suggest this remedy. The *nocturnal* aggravation should be one of our most prominent indications, and this will show itself in the character and intensity of the *pains, both in and around the eye.* The general condition of the patient will assist greatly in deciding our choice.

Nux vom. Disseminate choroiditis occurring in persons addicted to the use of stimulants, also when atrophic changes are even far advanced, Nux often seems to materially improve the degree of vision. The eyes are especially weak and *sensitive to light in the morning.* Gastric derangements and other constitutional symptoms are of great importance in selecting this drug.

Phosphorus. Both serous and disseminate choroiditis have been benefited, especially when accompanied by *photopsias and chromopsias of various shapes and colors* (red predominating). We find in the proving of Phosphorus, that it has produced *hyperœmia of the choroid*, and experience shows that it is often adapted to this condition. When sexual excesses seem to be the cause of the trouble, this remedy is indicated. The optic nerve and even retina may show decided hyperæmia. Black spots pass before the vision, and bright light, natural or artificial is injurious, while the eyes seem *better in the twilight.* Particularly suitable to lean slender persons, especially if complicated with cough, etc.

Prunus spin. Inflammation of the choroid, either with or without iritic or retinal complication. Haziness of the vitreous and the other common symptoms of the disease are present, but the characteristic indication will be found in the *pain which is usually severe as if the eyeball were being pressed asunder, or else sharp shooting and cutting through the eye and corresponding side of the head, or crushing in character.*

Pulsatilla. Hyperæmia of the choroid or sub-acute cases of choroiditis, occurring in women of a mild, tearful, yielding disposition and when accompanied by amenorrhœa, also in tea drinkers who are subject to neuralgic headaches. Eye symptoms not characteristic. (See Pulsatilla.)

Sulphur. Chronic cases of choroiditis, especially if traceable to the suppression of an eruption or if occurring in a strumous subject. *Sharp darting pains* are usually present. Often assists in clearing the vitreous and completing a cure, after other remedies have been used with advantage. The hemeralopia found in some cases may be relieved. For further indications see Sulphur.

In addition to the above, the following remedies have also been employed with favorable results. Acon. (first stage), Arsen. (dissem.), Colocy. (serous), Hepar, Ipecac. (serous), Psor. (serous), Ruta. (dissem.), Sil. (dissem.), Sol. nig. (dissem).

CHOROIDITIS SUPPURATIVA (PANOPHTHALMITIS.)

Our first endeavor should be to save the eye if possible, and with this end in view any exciting cause must be removed. If, for instance, it be due to a swollen cataractous lens this must be extracted, if to an orbital abscess this must be opened, or if a foreign body is found to be the cause, as frequently the case, we must try to remove it if possible, unless it is too deep within the eye, when it is far better to enucleate, except when the inflammatory process is very pronounced, when experience shows that it is advisable to wait until the severity of the symptoms have subsided, before we undertake the operation, but if a foreign body be present within the ball, we strongly recommend the enucleation of the eye after the inflammation has been subdued, for there is always danger of sympathetic irritation of the other eye.

For the disease itself, in the first stage, cold or ice compresses may be used with advantage, but if the pain be very severe in and around the eye, especially if suppuration has commenced, more benefit will usually be gained from warm applications, either dry or moist. Atropine may be of advantage early in palliating the pain, etc.

If the pain is very severe and the tension increased, paracentesis or an iridectomy will be found of service. If, however, suppuration has far advanced, so as to destroy the eye and the pain is intense, it is best to make a deep incision at once and employ hot fomentations, (a solution of Calendula).

Aconite. *First stage* accompanied by high fever, much thirst, etc. *Eyelids red, swollen, hot and dry*, and much pain in the eye.

Apis. *Lids œdematous, conjunctiva chemosed, stinging pains* through the eye. Drowsiness, and absence of thirst usually accompany.

Arsenic. If the patient is very *restless* and *thirsty*, with œdema of the lids and conjunctiva, with severe burning pain. Arsenicum cases are similar to Rhus, though the former does not compare with the latter in degree of usefulness.

Hepar. *After suppuration* has begun. *Eye very sensitive to touch* and the *pains severe* and *throbbing ameliorated by warm applications.*

Phytolacca. Of service, especially if of traumatic origin. *Lids very hard, red and swollen*, conjunctiva chemosed and pus in the interior of the eye. Pains quite severe.

Rhus tox. The most commonly indicated remedy in panophthalmitis, whether it be of traumatic origin or not. Is useful in nearly every stage of the disease, though is particularly adapted to the first. The *lids are œdematously swollen* and spasmodically closed, and upon opening them a profuse gush of tears pours out. The *conjunctiva is chemosed*, forming a wall around the cornea, which may be slightly hazy. The iris may be swollen, pupil contracted and aqueous cloudy, while the pain in and around the eye is often severe, especially at night and upon any change in the weather. A rheumatic diathesis, and if caused from exposure to wet or cold would suggest Rhus.

Asafœt., Bell., Merc., Sulph., and others may rarely and in certain stages be useful.

CHORIO-RETINITIS.

Compare therapeutics of Choroiditis and Retinitis.

SCLEROTICO-CHOROIDITIS POSTERIOR.

(Posterior Staphyloma.)

As myopia always accompanies this disorder of the fundus, the proper selection of glasses should receive our first attention, the greatest care being taken that they are not too strong. We should next warn the patient against overuse of the eyes, especially for near objects, and also to always avoid stooping or bending forward, when using the eyes at near work, as this tends to increase the venous congestion, thus serving to accelerate the progress of the disease. These patients should, therefore, sit erect with head thrown back, when reading and with back to the light, so that the page will be illuminated and the eyes not subjected to the bright glare of the light. The work or book should not be brought nearer as the eye becomes fatigued, but be laid aside until the eyes are thoroughly rested. If the patient complains of dazzling from the bright light, as is often the case, either blue or smoke glasses may be allowed. In aggravated cases they should be required to abstain from all near work.

The constant and continued use of *atropine* for a long time has been found advantageous in some instances.

Belladonna. Sclero-choroiditis posterior *with flushed face and throbbing congested headaches.* The eye appears hyperæmic externally as well as internally; the *optic nerve and whole fundus are seen congested.* Opacities may be present in the vitreous, photopsias and chromopsias are sometimes observed. The eyes are *quite sensitive to light.*

Crocus. Posterior staphyloma with pain extending from the eye to the top of the head, also a pain in the left eye darting to the right. Sensation of cold wind blowing across the eyes, (Fluoric ac.).

Mercurius. Syphilitic dyscrasia. Eyes red and irritable. Pains in and around the eye always *worse at night.* Artificial light is especially hurtful. General symptoms.

Phosphorus. Fundus hyperæmic, muscæ volitantes and flashes of light before the vision, etc.

Prunus spin. Staphyloma posticum, accompanied by *pains in ball as if pressed asunder, or sharp and shooting, in and around the eye.* Vitreous hazy and vessels of the fundus injected.

Spigelia. When accompanied by *sharp stabbing pains* through the eye and around it, often commencing at one point and then seeming to radiate in every direction.

Thuya. Is one of our most important remedies in all *inflammatory conditions of the sclera*, especially occurring in *strumous or syphilitic subjects.* The globe may be quite sensitive to touch and the photophobia is usually marked.

Carbo veg., Lyco., Kali iod., Physostigma, Ruta and Sulph., are also remedies to be borne in mind.

TUMORS OF THE CHOROID.

Tumors of the choroid are as a rule malignant in character, and therefore necessitate the enucleation of the eye as soon as recognized. Remedies that are recommended for sarcoma, carcinoma, etc., in other portions of the body might be tried, though delay in removing the eye is unwarranted.

RUPTURE OF THE CHOROID AND HEMORRHAGE.

The latter is the most common symptom that demands our attention in the treatment of the choroid, though we may have hemorrhages arising spontaneously, or from inflammatory changes, etc., etc.

The remedies chiefly called for, will be *Arn.*, Bell., China, Crotalus, Hamamelis, *Lach.*, Phos., etc. For special indications refer to retinitis apoplectica.

If there is hyperæmia or inflammation of the choroid present, our treatment will be guided by the rules laid down under choroiditis.

GLAUCOMA.

(*The Arthritic Ophthalmia of older writers.*)

Thanks to the genius of von Graefe, for the grandest discovery in ophthalmic science, the value of *iridectomy* in glaucoma. By the majority of the dominant school, iridectomy is considered the only true curative treatment for this affliction, and Homœopathy should by no means cast this important aid aside, but, upon the other hand, place it at the head of our remedial agents. We do not consider it the only measure we possess, to combat this terrible malady, for we have several drugs that have proved beneficial in staying the progress of the disease, especially in its incipiency, but when the premonitory stage has passed and there is no period of remission between the attacks, no physician is justified, in delaying to perform an iridectomy. This may be laid down as a rule, though there are exceptional cases, in which the operation does harm or proves of no service, as in the hemorrhagic form, though this should not deter us from operating, unless the hemorrhagic tendency is well marked, when we should first give our remedies a thorough trial.

Sclerotomy, myotomy and other operative measures are recommended, though none of them can as yet be compared to a large iridectomy, as a curative agent.

In the premonitory stage, as has already been said, our endeavor should be to cure by the aid of our drugs, which may be done in many cases, if we take into consideration the constitutional disturbances which co-exist with or cause the intraocular trouble, as gout, rheumatism, hemorrhoids, menstrual difficulties, etc. The habits of our patient should also receive careful attention. The excessive use of stimulants, either alcohol or tobacco, or any exhaustive mental or physical labor must be strictly forbidden. Only moderate use of the eyes should be allowed in any case, and during the attacks, or when they follow each other in rapid succession, complete rest is necessary. Bright light, either natural or artificial, should be avoided, or the eyes protected by colored glasses. The diet should be good and nutritious, particularly in elderly persons, and all indigestible substances or stimulants forbidden.

Belladonna. Often of benefit in relieving the severe pains of glaucoma, especially if accompanied by throbbing headache, flushed face, etc. The eyes are injected, pupils dilated, fundus hyperæmic, and pain both in and around the eye, varying greatly in character, though usually seems to be deep and of a pressing nature; sometimes, as if the eye were being torn out, or again, as if pressed into the head, etc. The eyes feel hot, dry and stiff, as if they might protrude. (Care must be taken to avoid the use of *atropine*, when glaucoma is suspected.)

Bryonia. On account of its action in serous inflammations in general, this remedy has been given with benefit in glaucoma. The eyes feel full as if pressed out, often associated with sharp shooting pains through the eye and head. *The eyes feel sore to touch and on moving them in any direction.* The usual concomitant symptoms help in deciding us in the selection.

Cedron. For the relief of the pains of glaucoma, when they are severe and *shooting along the course of the supra-orbital nerve.*

Colocynth. Of excellent service in relieving the pains of glaucoma when of a severe, burning, aching, sticking, *cutting* character in the eye and around, always *relieved by firm pressure* and by walking in a warm room, aggravated by rest at night and upon stooping.

Phosphorus. Fundus hyperæmic and hazy, halo around the light, and various lights and colors flashing before the eyes, especially when found in tall, slender patients.

Prunus spin. *Pain severe, crushing* in the eye *as if pressed asunder*, or *sharp shooting through the eye and corresponding side of the head* (Spig.). Aqueous and vitreous hazy, fundus hyperæmic.

Rhododendron. Incipient glaucoma, with much pain in and around the eye, periodic in character and *always worse just* *before a storm, ameliorated after the storm commences.* (Examine case under Rhodo., Part I.)

Spigelia. *Pains sharp and stabbing through the eye and head,* worse on motion and at night.

Our range of drugs will be extensive in this affection, as we must take into consideration all the general symptoms to make a sure prescription. Those remedies we have just mentioned have been most often called for in the cases we have met, though the following are also reported to have been found useful:—Arn., Ars., Aur., Cham., Cocc., Collin., Con., Crot. tig., Gels., Ham. v., Kali iod., Macrotin, Merc., Nux, Phyto., Sulph. and Val. of Zinc.

OPTIC NERVE AND RETINA.

NEURITIS AND RETINITIS.

(*Including Hyperœmia of the Optic Nerve and Retina.*)

Hyperæmia of the retina frequently depends upon some anomaly in the accommodation or refraction of the eye, which should be corrected by suitable glasses, after which the retina returns to its normal condition.

Rest is our most important aid in all cases, whether inflammatory or only hyperæmic, and the more complete (especially in neuritis, or retinitis), the better for the patient. They should be instructed to abstain from all use of the eyes, particularly by artificial light. Some authors, as Stellwag, and others, recommend the confinement of the patients in a darkened room, and the employment of a bandage, thus keeping all light away from the eye for some time, when they should gradually become accustomed to bright light. Such severe measures are, however, not required, except in extreme cases. It is better to allow moderate exercise in the open air, taking care that the eyes are properly protected from the irritating influence of bright light, by the use of either blue or smoke glasses.

Proper hygienic rules, according to the nature of the case, demand our most careful attention.

Belladonna. One of our most common remedies for both hyperæmia and inflammation of the optic nerve and retina. *The retinal vessels will be found enlarged and tortuous*, particularly the veins, while a *blue or bluish-gray film* often seems to overspread the fundus (œdema). *Extravasations of blood* may be numerous or few in number. *The optic disk is swollen*, and outlines ill defined. The vision is of course deteriorated. The pains are usually of an *aching*, dull character, though may be throbbing and severe, often accompanied by *throbbing*, *congested headaches*, with visibly beating carotids, flushed face, etc.

Phosphenes of every shape and hue are often observed. Decided *sensitiveness to light.* The eyes feel *worse in the afternoon* and evening, when all the symptoms are aggravated. Externally the eye may present no abnormal appearance, though generally seems weak; is injected and irritable (often with a red conjunctival line along the margins of the lids).

Bryonia. Serous retinitis or hyperæmia, with a bluish haze before the vision, and severe, *sharp pain* through the eye and over it. Eyes feel full, and *sore on motion* or to touch. Great heat in the head, aggravated by stooping.

Cactus. Retinal congestions, especially if heart troubles are present.

Conium. Fundus some congested, and accompanied by *much photophobia*, ciliary muscle weak.

Mercurius. Retinitis with marked nocturnal aggravation and *sensitiveness of the eyes to the glare of a fire.* Congested conditions of the fundus found in those who work at a forge, or over fires. Concomitant symptoms will assist us in the selection.

Nux vom. Retinitis occurring with gastric disturbances, especially in drunkards. The eye indications vary, but are usually *aggravated in the morning.*

Phosphorus. Both hyperæmia and inflammation of the optic nerve and retina are often benefited by this drug. The retina is congested and optic nerve hyperæmic. Photopsies and chromopsies, as halo around the light, are often present. Dimness of vision, and muscæ volitantes. Eyeballs may be sore on motion, and pain may extend from eyes to the top of the head. Photophobia may be present or absent.

Pulsatilla. When dependent upon *menstrual difficulties* (delayed or suppressed menstruation), or to a suppression of acne of the face, disorders of the stomach, etc. (See case reported under Puls., Part I.)

In addition to the above the following remedies have been recommended, and employed with benefit in rare cases, or as intercurrent remedies: Acon., Ars., Aurum, Collin., Con., Crocus, Gels., Kali iod., Kali mur., Lach., Leptan., Macrot., Spig., Sulph., and Zinc.

RETINITIS SYPHILITICA.

Asafœtida. When accompanied by *severe boring, burning pains above the brows*, especially at night; also if there is pain in the balls from within outwards, ameliorated by pressure (reverse of Aurum).

Aurum. Especially after *overdosing with iodide of potash or mercury*, and if accompanied by detachment of the retina. Eye sensitive to touch, and pain in and around, often seeming to be deep in the bones. A general syphilitic dyscrasia is perceptible in the constitutional symptoms which govern our selection of Aurum.

Kali iod. For syphilitic retinitis, this should be one of the first remedies thought of, especially if there is choroideal complication, though the chief indications for its use will be furnished by the general condition of the patient.

Mercurius. Especially the remedy for this form of inflammation of the retina. The solubis or corrosivus are more commonly employed, though the other preparations are also useful when special indications point to their use. The retina will be found hazy, congested, and often complicated with an inflammatory condition of the choroid or neighboring tissues. The eye is particularly sensitive to artificial light, and *nocturnal aggravation of all the symptoms* is always present. More or less pain is experienced both in and around the eye, especially during the evening and after going to bed. The syphilitic taint will be perceptible in various ways, that will indicate Merc.

Other anti-syphilitic remedies may be useful, given according to general indications, or we may find a remedy recommended for the other forms of retinitis serviceable in this variety, when particular indications are present.

RETINITIS ALBUMINURICA.

The principal treatment should be directed to the kidneys, the primary seat of the disease, and such hygienic and dietetic measures adopted as are recommended for Bright's disease. Benefit has been obtained from keeping the patient quiet in bed, and upon a low or skim milk diet.

Apis. Œdematous swelling of the lids and general dropsical condition. Patient very drowsy, little thirst and scanty urine.

Arsenicum. Patient restless at all times, especially at night after midnight, great thirst for small quantities. Urine scanty and albuminous.

Gelsemium. Retinitis albuminurica occurring during pregnancy. White patches and extravasations of blood in the retina. Dimness of vision appears suddenly. Serous infiltration into the vitreous making it hazy, is sometimes observed. The patient is thirstless and albumen is found in the urine.

Kalmia. Nephritic retinitis accompanied by much pain in the back as if it would break, etc.

Merc. corr. Has been more extensively used in *albuminuric retinitis* than any other remedy. The results are especially favorable when pregnancy appears to be the exciting cause of the difficulty.

As hemorrhages are usually found in the retina in this form of inflammation, compare the remedies recommended for retinitis apoplectica.

Hepar, Kali acet., Plumb. and Phos., have either been used or are highly recommended for this condition of the eye. In fact any remedy applicable to the disease of the kidney will often prove of service in the eye complication.

RETINITIS LEUCÆMIA.

The treatment must be directed to the relief of the cause, leucocythæmia.

RETINITIS APOPLECTICA.

Arnica. Retinal hemorrhages, particularly if of traumatic origin.

Belladonna. Apoplexy of the retina, especially when arising from or accompanied by congested headaches. Suppressed menstruation may be the cause of the difficulty. The retina and optic nerve will be found inflamed and congested.

Crotalus. In the snake poisons we possess our chief agents for producing absorption of extravasations of blood into the retina. Crotalus is one of these which have been used with advantage, though not as frequently as the following:—

Lachesis. From its use we have seen hemorrhages into the retina speedily disappear, and the accompanying inflammation rapidly diminish. It is very commonly called for when no characteristic symptoms are present, with the exception of the pathological changes. The retina and perhaps optic nerve are inflamed and congested, while throughout the swollen retina may be observed, extravasations of blood of various ages and sizes.

Phosphorus. In a hemorrhagic diathesis, when the concomitant indications point to its selection.

ISCHÆMIA RETINÆ.

When the anæmic condition of the retina is complete (vision entirely lost), paracentesis or iridectomy to diminish the intraocular tension becomes necessary. We sometimes observe a partial anæmia of the optic nerve and retina, associated with and dependent upon general anæmia. These cases should be treated by the administration of those medicines indicated by the general condition of the patient, as Calc., China, Ferrum, Phos., Puls., etc.

Agaricus has cured when accompanied by a tendency towards chorea.

HYPERÆSTHESIA RETINÆ.

If dependent upon any anomaly of refraction, the proper glass must first be prescribed.

In rare, severe cases it may be necessary to confine the patient to a dark room and then gradually accustom them to the light. Though usually it is better to advise plenty of exercise in the open air, having the eyes protected by smoke or blue glasses or shade. Especial attention must be paid to the general health of the patient.

Belladonna. *Hyperæsthesia of the retina*, particularly if dependent upon some anomaly of refraction. *Eyes very sensitive to light;* cannot bear it, as it produces such aching and pain in the eye and even headache. Flashes of light and sparks observed before the vision. The eye symptoms as well as the headache, are usually aggravated in the afternoon and evening.

Conium. *Over sensitiveness of the retina to light*, especially if accompanied with asthenopic symptoms so that he cannot read long without the letters running together, with pain deep in the eye. Excessive photophobia but fundus normal in appearance. Photopsia.

Lactic acid. Hyperæsthesia of the retina, with steady aching pain in and behind the eyeball.

Natrum mur. Especially in chlorotic females when there is great photophobia, together with muscular asthenopia. Some conjunctival injection with lachrymation. *Eyes feel stiff and ache on moving them or on reading.* Letters run together on attempting to read. Sticking, throbbing headache in the temples.

Nux vom. When the *photophobia is excessive in the morning* and better as the day advances.

Macrotin. Angell considers Macrotin more widely serviceable than any other one remedy.

Merc. sol. Eyes more sensitive to artificial light and in the evening.

Tartar em. Photophobia, especially in scrofulous subjects. Recommended highly for over sensitiveness of the retina by some.

A host of other remedies which produce marked photophobia, or are indicated by the general symptoms and cachexia of the patient, may be called for in this disorder, as Acon., China, Gels., Hep., Hyos., Ignat., Puls., Sulph., etc.

DETACHMENT OF THE RETINA.

If the retina has been detached, for any great length of time, very little can be done to restore the vision, but if seen early the prognosis is much more favorable.

If taken in the first stage, within a short time after the detachment has occurred, the patient should be confined to his bed, chiefly on his back and the eyes bandaged. This is of great importance in recovery. If it is impossible to confine the patient to his room, he must be warned to avoid all use of his eyes, and to keep as quiet as possible. If he must be out in the light, the eyes must be protected by darkly colored glasses. In many cases the constant use of atropine is of advantage, as it prevents accommodation and thus keeps the eye and tissues more quiet.

Operations to allow the escape of the fluid, both into the vitreous and externally are employed, but only temporary relief is usually obtained in this manner. It may, however, be advisable in some instances.

Apis. Fluid beneath the retina. Pressive pain in the lower part of the ball, with flushed face and head. Stinging pains through the eye. Œdematous swelling of the lids, etc.

Aurum. Has been used successfully, in many cases of amotio retinæ. Especially adapted to those cases which follow over-dosing by potash or mercury. The symptom under Aurum, which suggests its use is as follows: "Upper half of vision as if covered by a black body, lower half visible." The choroid or retina is usually inflamed and opacities are seen in the vitreous, giving rise to the "blacks" complained of by the patient.

Digitalis. Adapted to the general pathological condition and has this common symptom of detachment of the retina. "As if the upper half of vision were covered by a dark cloud, evenings on walking." Benefit has been seen from its use.

Gelsemium. Is one of our most prominent remedies for serous infiltration beneath the retina, especially if resulting from choroiditis with haziness of the vitreous and some pain. A bluish haze or wavering, is also often observed.

Ars., Bry., Hep., Kali iod., Merc., and *Rhus* are also remedies to be thought of for this condition.

ATROPHY OF THE OPTIC NERVE AND RETINA.

In true atrophy of the optic nerve very little can be done to restore vision, though we are often able to check its progress, by the selection of appropriate remedies, as indicated by general constitutional symptoms.

Electricity is reported to have been followed by some success.

The hypodermic injection of strychnia is the chief remedy of the old school, and has been used with marked advantage in some instances. (*Nux vom.* has been followed by more favorable results in our hands than any other drug.)

AMBLYOPIA POTATORUM ET NICOTIANA.

The first and chief point to be attended to, will be the cutting off of the use of all liquors and tobacco immediately, or the reduction of their use to a minimum. After which such remedies should be employed, as are found necessary to restore the whole system to its natural tone.

Arsenic. Seems especially adapted to loss of vision, dependent upon the use of tobacco.

Nux vom. Has been and probably always will be, the most important and most commonly called for remedy in this trouble, and the results following its use are often marvellous. There are no marked eye symptoms in this disease, and therefore nothing to guide us to this drug, with the exception of the cause.

AMAUROSIS AND AMBLYOPIA.

A great many cases are to be found on record, in which the diagnosis of amaurosis or amblyopia was made, though in all probability the great majority were not true instances of the above disorders, but of some intra-ocular disease which might have been recognized by the aid of the ophthalmoscope. Therefore due allowance must be made in all those cases, in which remedies produced such marvellous cures.

In the treatment both of amaurosis and amblyopia, we are compelled to rely chiefly upon internal medication; we must therefore see that our remedies are very carefully selected. As the eye indications are "nil" we must prescribe wholly upon the general symptoms and in doing this the cause of the trouble often furnishes us a valuable indication.

The following remedies are reported to have cured; for special indications refer to each remedy in Part I: Acon., Alumina, Ammon. gum., Arn., Ars., Aur. jod. and mur., Baryta carb., *Bell.*, Bovista, Calc., Chel., China., Crotal., Cyclam., Elaps., Gels., Hep., Ignat., Kali acet., Lyco., Merc., Nat. mur., *Phos.*, Puls., Ruta grav., Santon., Sep., Sil., Sulph., Thuya, Zinc.

EMBOLISM OF THE CENTRAL ARTERY OF THE RETINA.

Vision may in exceptional cases, return without any treatment, though it is better to give those remedies, that seem to be constitutionally required.

By reference to *Opium* a case will be found described, in which a cure was effected; whether or not this was due to the Opium administered, is a question.

HEMIOPIA.

Half vision is usually only a symptom of some deep disorder of the eye, but as it is sometimes the only symptom to be found, we will mention those remedies appropriate to it. (It must be remembered that this is often due to intra-cranial tumors or other troubles which are irremediable.)

Upper half of vision invisible: *Aurum* and *Dig.*

Right half of vision invisible: *Cyclamen*, *Lith. carb.* and *Lyco.*

Vertical hemiopia (either half invisible) *Bovista*, *Calc. carb.*, *Chin. sulph.*, *Lobel. inf.*, *Mur. ac.*, *Nat. mur.*, *Sep.*, and *Viola od.*

HEMERALOPIA.

In the treatment of night blindness, rest and protection of the eyes from bright light are first required. After which such constitutional remedies, as are necessary to restore the general health.

There are, however, certain drugs which are especially applicable to this condition of the eye and from which great benefit has been derived. The special indications are few and can be found by reference to each drug, where cases are described: Arg. nit., Bell., China, *Hyos.*, Lyco., Puls., *Ranunculus bulb.*, Stram., Sulph., and Verat.

NYCTALOPIA.

Is rarely observed in this country though would suggest, besides careful protection of the eyes, from bright light and general hygienic measures, the use of *Phos.* as the remedy most nearly adapted to this condition.

TUMORS OF THE RETINA.

These are usually gliomatous in character, and the only treatment that is in any degree effectual, as far as known, is *enucleation of the eye*, taking care to divide the optic nerve as far back toward the optic foramen as possible.

LENS.

CATARACT.

A large number of cases are to be found in our literature, in which the internal administration of a few doses of the properly selected remedy has worked a wonderful cure of cataract, but the great majority of these must be taken "cum grano salis," and put aside with the remark "mistaken diagnosis."

We are, however, certain, that by a careful selection of drugs according to the homœopathic law, and by continuing the use for a long period, we may succeed in a large proportion of cases, in checking the progress of the disease, and are often enabled to clear up a portion of the diffuse haziness, thus improving vision to a certain extent. But after degeneration of the lens fibres has taken place, no remedy will be found of avail, in restoring its lost transparency and improving the sight. We must then, providing the vision is seriously impaired, and it is senile or hard cataract, wait until it has become mature, when the lens should be extracted.

The operations employed are various, nearly every surgeon having a modification of his own; they also vary according to the condition of the eye and the character of the cataract. The operations are already well described in our standard text books on the eye.

The medical treatment will consist of the selection of remedies according to the constitutional symptoms observed in the patient, for the objective indications are entirely or nearly absent, as we cannot yet decide from the appearance of an opaque lens what remedy is required.

The drugs found below, have been verified by us, as having arrested the progress of the cataract. Baryta carb., Calc., CAUST., Lyco., *Magn. carb.*, PHOS., SEPIA, *Sil.* and Sulph.

DISLOCATION OF THE LENS.

The treatment of a dislocated lens varies greatly, according to the condition of the eye and the nature of the displacement. It is only by operative interference, that favorable results can be obtained, except we may be able to relieve pain by the use of atropine, or by internal medication. (See ciliary neuralgia.)

VITREOUS HUMOR.

HYALITIS.

Inflammation of the vitreous is usually complicated with some other severe inflammation of the fundus, as irido-cyclitis, irido-choroiditis, etc. Therefore, for treatment, compare that recommended for the above diseases. A foreign body might be mentioned as the most common cause of this disorder, in which case enucleation of the eye is the only practicable remedy.

OPACITIES OF THE VITREOUS.

This condition is usually only a symptom, or a result of some deep-seated disturbance in the internal structures, and, therefore, the primary disorder requires our attention at first. Where it is the result of an inflammatory process, or, when it occurs spontaneously or independently, there are certain remedies which have been followed by excellent results, and are to be thought of, such as: Arn., Bell., Ham. v., Kalmia, Kali iod., Lach., Lyco., Merc., Phos., Prunus, Sil., Sol. nig., Sulph., etc.

Electricity is reported to have benefited.

Fixed opacities have occasionally been torn through with a fine needle and the vision improved.

FOREIGN BODIES AND CYSTICERCI IN THE VITREOUS.

The treatment, employed for injuries of the eye, may prove of service in allaying the inflammatory symptoms, after the introduction of a foreign body; but, as a rule in all cases, in which a foreign body is present in the vitreous humor, *enucleate the eye as soon as possible*, in order that the other eye may not be endangered through sympathy. In rare cases, occurring in intelligent persons, who live near us, we may allow the eye to remain, if the foreign body has become encysted and is producing no irritation, directing them to have it immediately removed, upon the first appearance of any sympathetic irritation.

If a cysticercus is found in the vitreous, only operative measures are of any avail.

REFRACTION AND ACCOMMODATION.

MYOPIA.

Nearsightedness is an anomaly of refraction which requires special and careful attention, as its tendency is to constantly progress until it may terminate in complete blindness.

There are four points in the treatment of Myopia which require our consideration, as follows: 1. To prevent its further development and the occurrence of secondary disturbances. 2. By means of suitable glasses to render the use of the eye easier and safer. 3. To remove any existing muscular asthenopia. 4. To combat the secondary disturbances.

Our first and most important aim should be to check the progress of the myopia, and this we are able to do, providing the patient will adhere closely to the directions given. In the beginning we must ascertain the cause of the trouble, whether due to elongation of the antero-posterior axis of the ball, or to spasm of the ciliary muscle. In either case if the myopia is rapidly increasing, complete *rest* of the eyes, especially for near objects, is necessary, but if the increase is slow or nearly stationary, moderate use of the eyes may be allowed, with this condition, that they *avoid too strong convergence of the optic axis;* that is, whenever they use the eyes for near objects, either with or without glasses, to carry the object away as far as it can be seen distinctly, and not bring it near the eye, which is the tendency when the eyes become tired. It is also desirable that patients discontinue work, and rest the eyes from two to five minutes every half hour, more or less.

A *stooping position* will also promote the increase of myopia, particularly if posterior staphyloma is present, as an increased amount of blood is sent to the eye, which accelerates the inflammatory process going on within; therefore the patient must be advised to *sit as erect as possible*, and, if compelled to write, use a sloping desk. The light should be placed behind, shining over the shoulder upon the work, and not in front, directly in the eyes, as it would irritate and increase the inflammatory symptoms. When the bright light is very dazzling and annoying, colored glasses may be allowed. If antero-posterior elongation of the eyeballs be the cause of the myopia, the treatment, remedial and otherwise, recommended for sclerotico-choroiditis posterior should be followed.

Within the last two years spasm of the accommodation has been placed in the foremost rank, by many prominent oculists, as a cause for nearsightedness, making decided changes in the manner of treatment.

Calabar bean, employed internally, has been followed by favorable results in many cases of myopia, dependent upon spasm of the ciliary muscle, checking the progress of the disease, and often restoring a portion of the lost vision.

The constant use of a weak solution of *Atropine*, instilled into the eye for a long time, keeping the ciliary muscles at perfect rest, until they have recovered their normal tone, is frequently advantageously used, though the inconvenience experienced by the abnormal dilatation of the pupil, and loss of accommodation, often prevents its employment.

For further and special treatment, compare the section on spasm of the ciliary muscle. Marked attention should be paid to the general health of the patient, as well as to the eye.

Secondly. "By means of suitable glasses to render the use of the eye easier and safer." This might be properly considered under the first point, as it is of the greatest importance in preventing the development of myopia, that the proper spectacles be selected, and that only these be worn, for there is nothing that causes any existing nearsightedness to increase so rapidly as the use of improper glasses, especially if too strong, as they are liable to be. We can only give a few general rules regarding the selection of spectacles, when to advise their use and when to forbid.

The best general rule that can be given in prescribing spectacles for a myopic eye, though there are exceptional cases that it will not cover, is as follows: Never recommend the use of glasses for myopia if the patient can easily get along without them; but if found necessary, give the *weakest glass* that will render vision easy (though not usually perfect), and remove unpleasant symptoms. We very often prescribe glasses in myopia for distance, that will nearly neutralize the degree, but usually advise them not to wear them constantly, only employ them when they wish to see an object distinctly. Also give glasses, according to the general rule for reading music, or seeing objects two feet or more distant, with the injunction not to use them for any other distance. For reading or near vision, we rarely recommend glasses, unless the myopia is great, or muscular asthenopia is present, and the exceptions hereafter noted are absent, in which cases they may be allowed.

Many circumstances forbid the neutralization of the myopia, as follows: 1. If the degree of myopia is slight. 2. If the range of accommodation is contracted. 3. If the acuteness of vision is materially decreased. 4. If the nature of the work does not render them necessary.

Thirdly. "To relieve any existing muscular asthenopia." This can be done by suitable concave glasses, the use of prisms, tenotomy of the external rectus, and the selection of the indicated remedy. (See section on asthenopia.)

Fourthly. "To combat the secondary disturbances." These, whatever they may be, must be treated according to the principles laid down in corresponding sections.

PRESBYOPIA.

This condition is only physiological, and therefore requires no treatment, with the exception of the selection of the proper spectacles. As a rule give the glass with which they see the easiest and most distinctly, at from twelve to sixteen inches. No glasses are required for distance, except occasionally, in very old people, when a slight degree of hypermetropia may develope.

Prescribe glasses for presbyopia just as soon as any difficulty or inconvenience is experienced in seeing near objects, as, instead of increasing the amount of far-sightedness, as many suppose, it tends to prevent its increase, and relieves all asthenopic symptoms.

It must always be borne in mind that a rapid increase of presbyopia is a prominent symptom of glaucoma, in which, of course, glasses should not be given, but other measures resorted to.

HYPERMETROPIA.

The first and most important indication, is the selection of proper convex glasses; in fact, this is the only treatment of this affection "per se," though the resulting symptoms of asthenopia, etc., may require further attention. Spectacles should be prescribed for hyperopia *immediately* upon the appearance of asthenopic symptoms. In selecting these glasses we should first determine the degree of manifest hyperopia (Hm.), by finding the strongest convex glass with which the patient can see perfectly, at a distance (No. 20 at twenty feet.) This glass which corresponds to or neutralizes Hm., is usually the one which the patient requires for near vision, though in some cases they cannot bear as strong a glass as this to commence with, while in others it is also necessary to neutralize a portion of the latent hyperopia (Hl.) Many oculists recommend the neutralization of all of Hm. and one-fourth of Hl., but these glasses are usually found too strong for the patient.

The best general rule to follow, is, to give the *strongest convex glass* with which the patient can read distinctly and easily, for a length of time, at the usual distance for near vision.

As a rule, glasses should not be advised for distant vision, unless the hyperopia is relative or absolute, when their use becomes necessary.

Asthenopia, both accommodative and muscular, though more frequently the former, arise from hyperopia. Both are, however, relieved by the proper selection of convex glasses, and often cured by this measure alone, but if some weakness of the muscles remain, special treatment is required, as can be seen by reference to the section devoted to asthenopia.

A measure of the greatest importance for the relief of asthenopic symptoms, dependent upon hyperopia, is *systematic exercise of the eyes with convex glasses*, as first recommended by Dr. Dyer. For instance, give the proper convex glass and advise its use for reading, every morning and afternoon, at a regular time, for from three to ten minutes, according to the amount of asthenopia, and increase the time one minute each day, as long as it can be done without pain.

The treatment of strabismus convergens, or any other complication, can be found under appropriate heads.

ASTIGMATISM.

The only treatment for regular astigmatism consists in the careful selection of cylindrical glasses, either simple cylindrical, spherico-cylindrical, or by-cylindrical, according to the variety of astigmatism we have to deal with.

Irregular astigmatism is dependent upon irregular refraction of the lens or cornea, caused chiefly in the latter case by inflammatory changes. In these instances stenopaic spectacles may be necessary, or the performance of an iridectomy. Benefit may also be obtained from the use of drugs, as seem indicated by the appearance and condition of the eye. A case may be found under Sepia.

MUSCLES AND NERVES.

PARTIAL OR COMPLETE PARALYSIS OF THE MUSCLES OF THE EYE.

The treatment varies according to the nature of the cause which should always receive due consideration in the selection of the drug.

The prescription of prismatic glasses to which we sometimes resort, has in view the accomplishment of two objects. 1. To relieve the annoying diplopia by giving that prism which neutralizes the diplopia. 2. For the purpose of exercising the paralyzed muscle by using a weaker prism, thus nearly fusing the double images, when by the exercise of the will they may be brought together. Care must be taken in the latter case, however, not to use too weak or too strong a glass.

Electricity or galvanization is another very important aid in the cure of this disorder, either alone or in connection with the appropriate remedy.

As a last resort, a careful tenotomy of the opposing muscle may be performed, with or without advancement of the paralyzed muscle at the same time, according to the degree of deviation.

Arnica. Paralysis of the muscles resulting from a blow or injury.

Argentum nit. For weakness of the ciliary muscle or even paralysis of the accommodation, manifest advantage has been derived.

Causticum. Paralysis of the muscles resulting from *exposure to cold.* Has been especially successful in paralysis of the levator palpebræ superioris (ptosis), orbicularis and external rectus; thus its action is not found confined to any one nerve, but is useful in paralysis of any of the ocular muscles, if the particular cause and general indications are present.

Cuprum acet. Paralysis of the nervus abducentis. (See clinical application of Cuprum, Part I.)

Euphrasia. Paralysis of the muscles, particularly of the third part, when caused from exposure to cold and wet, especially if catarrhal symptoms of the conjunctiva, blurring of the eyes relieved by winking, etc., are present.

Gelsemium. Important in paralysis of the muscles, but general indications must furnish our chief guides in its selection.

Kali iodata. The iodide of potash is perhaps more commonly indicated than any other drug in paralysis of the muscles of *syphilitic origin.* (Appreciable doses are usually employed.)

Mercurius. Especially if of a syphilitic origin. (See Merc. prot., Part I.)

Nux vom. Paresis of the ocular muscles, particularly if made worse by the use of stimulants or tobacco.

Opium. Paralysis of the accommodation. (See Opium, Part I.)

Paris quad. Paralysis of the iris and ciliary muscle, with pain drawing from eye to back of the head; or pain as if the eyes were pulled into the head. Eyes sensitive to touch.

Phosphorus. Paralysis of the muscles caused from or accompanied by spermatorrhœa, sexual abuse, hemorrhoids, etc.

Physostigma ven. As a local application in partial or complete paralysis of the accommodation, has been employed with benefit.

Rhus tox. A remedy of great importance and often indicated. Paralysis of any of the ocular muscles resulting from *rheumatism* or *exposure to cold*, *wet weather*, getting the feet wet, etc. Causticum is very similar in its action, though is more especially adapted, we think, to those cases resulting from exposure to cold, dry weather.

Senega. Especially in want of power of the superior rectus or superior oblique, in which the *diplopia is relieved by bending the head backward.* The other muscles may be complicated in the trouble.

Spigelia. When associated with *sharp stabbing pains* through the eye and head.

Alumina, Aurum, Conium and Hyoscyamus, have also been used with advantage, as may other remedies if symptoms so indicate.

SPASM OF THE MUSCLES OF THE EYE.

(*Including nystagmus, blepharospasmus and spasms of the ciliary muscle.*)

Agaricus. Is the most commonly indicated of all our drugs for spasmodic affections of the muscles of the eye, particularly *spasm of the lids*, though has also been very useful in controlling the spasmodic action of the internal recti and the ciliary muscle. It is therefore a prominent remedy for myopia, dependent upon spasm of the accommodation, especially if associated with spasmodic affections of other muscles. *Twitchings of the lids*, varying from frequent winking to spasmodic closure of them; *chorea like spasm of the lids*, with general heaviness of them, constitute its chief sphere of action. *Twitchings of the balls*, with various sensations in and around them, chiefly pressing and aching. Eyeball sensitive to touch. The *spasmodic movements are absent during sleep but return on waking*, and are often transiently relieved by washing in cold water. Very little or no inflammatory action is present. Twitching in other parts of the body may often be found.

Atropine. The steady use of a weak solution of atropine to the eye for a long time has been followed by favorable results in spasm of the ciliary muscle.

Belladonna. If accompanied by headache and hyperæsthesia of the senses.

Cicuta. *See Strabismus.*

Hyoscyamus. Spasmodic action of the eyeballs.

Ignatia. Morbid nictitation occurring in nervous hysterical women.

Physostigma ven. In its proving there has been developed marked spasmodic action of the ciliary muscle and muscles of the lid. It has therefore been used with manifest advantage in these conditions, particularly the former; and as spasm of the ciliary muscle is frequently found in myopia, it should always be thought of in this anomaly of refraction. The patient cannot read long on account of this spasm and must bring the book near the eyes. There is also generally to be seen *twitchings in the lids and around the eyes* when Physostigma is required. The pupil is contracted.

Nux, Puls. and Sulph., have also been used with advantage, as may any of that class of remedies denominated our anti-spasmodics. (Compare Therapeutics of strabismus.)

STRABISMUS.

Careful distinction must be made between concomitant and paralytic squint, as the treatment materially varies. As strabismus convergens is frequently due to hyperopia, and strabismus divergens to myopia, we must always at first obtain the patient's refraction. If either be the cause, the ametropia should be neutralized, when, if the squint is recent and periodic in character, a cure may be effected by this means alone or in connection with internal medication. In recent cases advantage may be derived from careful and systematic exercise of the weaker muscle, either with or without prisms, especially if the squint is of the paralytic variety.

In true concomitant squint, after it has become permanent, we should perform tenotomy of the contracting muscle, and do it as *early as possible*, in order, that no sight be lost from non-use. Care must be taken, after the operation, to prescribe glasses, if an anomaly of refraction was the cause of the trouble, so that its return may be prevented, if possible.

Cicuta vir. Commonly indicated in strabismus convergens found in children, particularly, if of a spasmodic nature, or caused from convulsions, to which the child is subject.

Cyclamen. Reported to have cured strabismus, arising from convulsions, helminthiasis, falls, following measles, etc.

When helminthiasis has been the cause, Cina, Cyclamen., Sep., Spig. and Sulph. have cured. If due to spasms, convulsions, or any intra-cranial disorders, Agar., Bell., Hyos., Nux, Stram., Tabac., etc., would be first suggested to our minds.

Other remedies, reported to have cured cases, are as follows: Alumina, Aur., Calc., Chin., Sulph., Kali jod. and Phos.

In all cases we must determine the cause of the difficulty, if possible; for this, in connection with the general condition of the patient, will govern us in the selection of the remedy.

Compare treatment, given for both paralysis and spasm of the muscles of the eye.

ASTHENOPIA.

(*Accommodative and muscular.*)

In a great majority of instances the cause of asthenopia is due to some anomaly of refraction, we must, therefore, correct this by *suitable glasses*, before any headway can be made in the treatment; after which properly indicated remedies are of great service. Not rarely we find asthenopia dependent upon entirely different causes, as general muscular laxity, debilitating diseases, and many other constitutional disturbances; in which case our treatment should be directed to the primary seat of the trouble. After prescribing the proper spectacles in asthenopia, only a moderate use of the eyes should be encouraged, until the over-worked muscles have regained their normal tone. (Compare treatment of asthenopia under hypermetropio.)

In insufficiency of the internal recti muscles, besides the spherical glasses necessary to overcome the faulty construction of the eye, prisms may also be required, either to relieve any existing diplopia, and, at the same time, employ binocular vision, or used with a view of strengthening the weak muscle. Again we have observed favorable results from systematic exercise of the internal recti, at regular periods, by having the patient regard his finger or a ruler, while it is slowly carried far to the right and then to the left, or, by carrying it near and from the eye.

Galvanism has also proved of advantage in some cases.

As a last resort, careful tenotomy of the external recti may be performed.

Aconite. Asthenopia from overuse of the eyes. Lids spasmodically closed, and have a heavy feeling in them, while the eyes *feel very hot and dry* after using. Conjunctiva may be hyperæmic. Cold water may relieve temporarily the heat in the eyes.

Agaricus. Asthenopia especially muscular, if accompanied by *sudden jerks of the ball, twitching of the lids, etc.*

Apis. When accompanied by redness of the eyes, lachrymation and *stinging pains.*

Calcarea. Pale, flabby subjects inclined to grow fat, with coldness of the extremities and perspiration about the head. Eyes pain after using, and are generally worse in damp weather and from warmth.

Cinnabar. Asthenopia with *pain from the inner canthus, extending above or around the eye;* exit of supra-orbital nerve sore to touch.

Conium. A prominent remedy for asthenopia. Cannot read long without the letters running together; burning pain deep in the eye. *Inability to bear either light* or heat is rarely absent.

Euphrasia. Eyes irritable from overuse, with *blurring of the vision, relieved by winking.*

Ignatia. Asthenopia in nervous hysterical females, especially if dependent upon onanism.

Kalmia. When there is present a stiff, drawing sensation in the muscles upon moving the eyes (*Natr. mur.*)

Natrum mur. We have found no remedy oftener indicated in asthenopia—particularly muscular—than this. Cannot read only a short time before the letters run together, with aching in and around the eyes. *The muscles feel stiff and drawn, and ache on moving the eye in any direction.* On looking down, a sharp pain above the eye may be present. The eyes appear irritable, and after using they smart, itch and burn. They wish to keep the eyes firmly closed, and something pressed hard against them.

Phosphorus. Eyes ache on moving, and feel hot and painful after using. Bright light, either artificial or natural, aggravates the trouble, so that the patient is *better in the twilight.* Musci volitantes and photopsa are often observed.

Physostigma ven. Calabar bean, in solution, employed locally, is used and highly recommended at the present day, in asthenopia muscularis, by prominent oculists of the old school. Its constant use must be continued for weeks to effect a cure.

Rhododendron. Insufficiency of the internal recti muscles, with darting pains through the eyes and head, *always worse before a storm.*

Ruta grav. Ruta stands side by side with Natr. mur., in frequency of indication in asthenopia (especially accommodative). Aching in and *over the eyes*, with blurring of the vision after using or straining the eyes at fine work. The *eyes feel hot*, like balls of fire, appear irritable, and run water, especially along toward evening, after working all day. Ruta is more often indicated in accommodative asthenopia, and Natr. mur. in muscular.

Santonine. Has been recommended for asthenopia dependent upon anomalies of refraction.

Spigelia. When accompanied by *sharp, stabbing pains* through the eye and around it, extending back into the head.

Besides the above, the following remedies have also been used with advantage, though special indications have not been marked, as can be seen by reference to clinical description of the drugs: Alumina, Ammon. carb., Arn., Asarum, Bell., Carbo veg., Kali carb., Lith. carb., Macrot., Mangan., Nux, Petrol., Puls., Secale, Sepia, Sulph., and Tabac.

NEURALGIA CILIARIS.

Ciliary neuralgia is usually only a symptom of some disorder of the eye, but as it is occasionally found unassociated with any ocular trouble, we shall speak briefly of those remedies adapted to this condition.

Asafœtida. *Severe, boring, tearing pain over the eyes*, also intense burning in brows, especially at night.

Belladonna. *Orbital neuralgias*, especially of the infra-orbital nerve, with red face, hot head, throbbing headache, etc.

Atropine, used locally in the eye, often proves of decided benefit in allaying the severe pain in and around the eyes.

Bryonia. *Pains severe, sharp*, and shooting *through the eye, back into the head*, or *extending from the eye down to malar bone, and then back to occiput.* The seat of pain becomes sore to touch. *Moving the eyeball in any direction*, or the exertion of talking, walking, etc., *will aggravate the pain*, so that he wishes constantly to keep the eyes closed and at perfect rest.

Cedron. One of the first remedies to be thought of in *supra-orbital neuralgia. Pains severe, sharp and shooting, starting from one point over the eye* (generally left) *and extending along the branches of the supra-orbital nerve into the head.*

May extend to temples or occiput; often worse in the evening, on lying down, and before a storm.

China. *Intermittent ciliary neuralgia.* (See clinical description.) (*The Muriate of Quinine*, in appreciable doses, will often alleviate *intense pain in and around the eye*, when *periodic in character*, especially if of malarial origin, and accompanied by chills.)

Cimicifuga rac. *Severe aching* pains in the eye-balls, or in the temples, extending to eyes. *Sharp, shooting pains, from occiput through to eyes, or from the eyes to the top of the head.*

Generally worse in the afternoon and night, and relieved on lying down. (Macrotin has been employed in similar cases with benefit.)

Cinnabaris. *Pain commencing at internal canthus, and extending over or around the eye.*

Prunus spin. Commonly indicated, especially if the pain in the eye-ball be severe and crushing, *as if pressed asunder*, or if the pain is sharp and *shooting* in character, through the eye and corresponding side of the head. These *severe, sharp pains* may commence in various portions of the head, and extend around and in the eye.

Silicea. Ciliary neuralgia; darting pains through the eye and head, often seeming to commence at occiput and extending forward to eyes, caused from exposure to a draft of air, and *relieved by keeping the head warm.*

Spigelia. Is a grand remedy in controlling the severe ciliary pain arising from various eye troubles, or independent of any such disorder. The pains may intermit or not, and are usually of a *sharp, stabbing character*, either around the eye, or *extending* through the eye into the head; they often seem to commence *at one point and then radiate in different directions.*

The pains are usually worse at night and on motion. Besides the above, which are most characteristic, there are a great variety of pains which have been relieved by Spigelia, as can be seen by referring to the clinical action of the drug.

Many other remedies may be indicated and useful in alleviating the severe pain in and around the eyes, chief among which may be mentioned Carbol. ac., Cham., Chel., Comoclad., Crotal., Ign., Ipecac, Mez., Nat. mur., Phell., Plat., Sulph., and Thuya.

For special indications see the clinical application of the drugs.

www.ingramcontent.com/pod-product-compliance
Lightning Source LLC
LaVergne TN
LVHW010226110826
845151LV00004B/1199